"Richmond combines theory and practice into a singular work of clinical insight that is sure to prove indispensable in helping mental health professionals guide survivors of sexual trauma from pain to passion. The exercises at the end of each chapter are awesome!"

—**Ian Kerner**, codirector of the sex therapy program at the Institute For Contemporary Psychotherapy, and *New York Times* bestselling author of *She Comes First*

"Holly Richmond is a wealth of knowledge when it comes to trauma and sexual healing. Her writing is dynamic, loving, and affirming in a way all survivors of sexual trauma deserve. *Reclaiming Pleasure* will undoubtedly be an invaluable resource for both trauma survivors and practitioners like myself who work with these incredibly brave individuals."

—**Gigi Engle, ACS**, certified clinical sexologist, and author of *All the F*cking Mistakes*

"In her groundbreaking book, Holly Richmond promises stuck survivors cut off from integral parts of ourselves that we can—and *will*—experience desire, ecstasy, and eroticism again (or for the very first time). Then—and this part is important—she shows us *how*. A beautifully written must-read for survivors ready to thrive."

—**Linda Kay Klein**, author of *Pure*, and founder of Break Free Together

"Finally, a smart and truly helpful book for survivors who want to experience sexual pleasure, passion, and joy. These are your right, and Holly Richmond will help you access them."

—**Wednesday Martin, PhD**, #1 *New York Times*
bestselling author of *Untrue* and *Primates of Park Avenue*

"Holly Richmond manages to bridge information with heart, touching on subject matter that so many of us hide deep inside. She calls us all into the process of reclaiming pleasure, but also reclaiming ourselves in the process. I am thankful the world has this resource of a book, and the wise, impactful words of Holly Richmond."

—**Chinae Alexander**, social entrepreneur, content creator
at ChinaeAlexander, writer, speaker, and host of the
Press Send Podcast

"Blending both grounded theory and narrative, Holly Richmond's work, *Reclaiming Pleasure*, takes the taboo and forbidden topics like sexuality and violation into the light of clear understanding. Richmond provides invaluable vocabulary and nuanced definitions for the complicated but necessary conversations that guide survivors to behavior that ensures our thriving. As a survivor of childhood sexual abuse, *Reclaiming Pleasure* is both affirming and empowering and has facilitated life-altering healing"

—**Colin Bedell**, cosmopolitan astrologer, and
best-selling author

"Paving the way forward for survivors and those who love them, *Reclaiming Pleasure* is a doorway to vitality, freedom, and transformation. It gives vocabulary to the ideas and feelings many have but haven't yet been able to articulate. Reading it feels like going on a road trip with your best friend, wise mentor, and healing balm in one."

—**Mal Harrison**, executive director of The Center
for Erotic Intelligence

"I am thrilled to have the opportunity to endorse this insightful and much-needed book by Holly Richmond. Richmond gives high-quality and important information to help those who have experienced sexual trauma live a passionate and sex-positive life. The book is well written, easy to follow, and gives behavioral exercises that are valuable and easy to understand."

—**Rachel Needle, PsyD**, codirector of Modern Sex
Therapy Institutes, and licensed psychologist and
executive director at Whole Health Psychological Center

"Holly Richmond makes an invaluable contribution to the field of psychotherapy where trauma and sexuality do not usually intersect. Her book is the first to talk about going from sexual trauma to sexual triumph inclusive of sex-positive information. Without this, clients are left on their own without help to identify what sex and erotica is for them. This book provides a pathway for those interested in healing with a sexual health component."

—**Joe Kort, PhD, LMSW**, author of *Is My Husband
Gay, Straight, or Bi?*; and codirector of Modern Sex
Therapy Institutes

Reclaiming

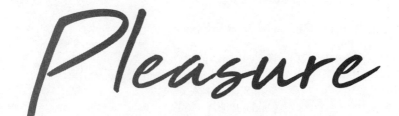

Pleasure

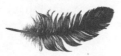

A SEX POSITIVE GUIDE for

MOVING PAST SEXUAL TRAUMA

& LIVING a PASSIONATE LIFE

HOLLY RICHMOND, PhD

New Harbinger Publications, Inc.

Publisher's Note

This publication is designed to provide accurate and authoritative information in regard to the subject matter covered. It is sold with the understanding that the publisher is not engaged in rendering psychological, financial, legal, or other professional services. If expert assistance or counseling is needed, the services of a competent professional should be sought.

NEW HARBINGER PUBLICATIONS is a registered trademark of New Harbinger Publications, Inc.

Distributed in Canada by Raincoast Books

In consideration of evolving American English usage standards, and reflecting a commitment to equity for all genders, 'they/them' is used in this book to denote singular persons.

Cover design by Amy Daniel; Acquired by Jennye Garibaldi; Edited by Mya Byrne

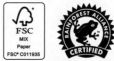

Library of Congress Cataloging-in-Publication Data

Names: Richmond, Holly, author.
Title: Reclaiming pleasure : a sex-positive guide for moving past sexual trauma and living a passionate life / Holly Richmond, PhD.
Description: Oakland, CA : New Harbinger Publication, [2021] | Includes bibliographical references.
Identifiers: LCCN 2021017860 | ISBN 9781684038428 (trade paperback)
Subjects: LCSH: Sexual abuse victims--Sexual behavior. | Sexual health. | Sex instruction.
Classification: LCC HV6625 .R53 2021 | DDC 362.88301/9--dc23
LC record available at https://lccn.loc.gov/2021017860

Printed in the United States of America

23   22   21

10   9   8   7   6   5   4   3   2   1   First Printing

This book is dedicated to all of the survivors who have courageously shared their heads and hearts— my greatest teachers and perpetual stars.

Thriving, a Manifesto

I will grow, flourish, prosper, and realize a goal despite—and because of—my circumstances.

Contents

Foreword

There is nothing wrong with you. Something happened to you.
That's different.

—Holly Richmond

Because this is a book about sexual trauma, you surely wish you did not need to read it. But here is what I promise you: this is a book you will be forever grateful you read. I hope you know that you are beyond brave for even picking this book up. Your willingness to open it reflects your commitment to your healing...or at least your curiosity about the potential for your healing.

I have spent the last two decades working as a licensed clinical psychologist, a professor, and a relationship expert. I have studied trauma and worked with survivors, and what I know for sure is that healing is a journey. *I also know for sure that Holly will be your competent and gentle guide on this journey.* Holly and I first crossed paths when we were both on faculty at an annual conference hosted by the iconic couples' therapist Esther Perel. When we introduced ourselves, I had that rare and wonderful sense I was meeting someone I had known for a long time. I was immediately struck by her warmth and humility. Then she took the stage to give her talk. She commanded this room full of hundreds of therapists and coaches—we hung on her every word. She shared stories about her many years of working with survivors of sexual trauma, moving seamlessly between science, stories, and skills. She was magnificent.

Holly lives, without apology or pretense, at the sacred intersection of kindness and expertise, the place from which she wrote *Reclaiming Pleasure*. Holly has what it takes to guide you on a journey into the most painful chapters of your life story, chapters you have potentially spent years avoiding. She provides you with:

- The *information* you have always needed and deserved—information about sexuality, trauma, and our wise and honest bodies.

- The *empathy* you have always needed and deserved—empathy that helps you move from ashamed to peaceful, from detached to alive, and from afraid to empowered.

- The *tools* you have always needed and deserved—tools that are scientifically proven to help you heal your trauma so you can stop feeling bad and start feeling good.

As Peter Levine said, "Trauma is not what happens to us, but what we hold inside in the absence of an empathic witness." Holly is your empathic witness. You are no longer alone.

In *Reclaiming Pleasure*, you will move through a three-step process of control, pleasure, and connection. Step one, *control*, anchors you in your body so you can feel safe and empowered. Step two, *pleasure*, returns you to sensation, expression, and presence so you can feel alive and aroused. Step three, *connection*, supports you as you open yourself to erotic intimacy with a partner. Holly's approach is sex-positive, which she defines this way: "*All sex is good sex as long as it's consensual and pleasurable.*" This book is at once personal and political, in all of the best ways!

Trauma science has taught us that healing is less about talking the talk and more about walking the walk. Healing trauma requires us to attend to our bodies, and Holly's training as a somatic psychologist infuses every page of *Reclaiming Pleasure*. This approach invites you into a profoundly compassionate relationship with your body and with the trauma-related symptoms your body may be experiencing. As Holly encourages, "Rather than asking yourself, 'What is wrong with me?' or 'Why can't I be normal?' ask your body and your symptoms, 'What are you trying to protect me from?' and 'How do you think you are keeping me safe?'" There is such a peace that arises when we stop doing battle with our bodies and begin to listen to them instead.

In order to maximize your healing, you will need to work through this book slowly. I invite you to take time completing the exercises that Holly has lovingly infused along the way. Because healing is a holistic process, the exercises woven throughout the book will ensure that you are engaging your mind, your emotions, and your body. The beauty of a book like this is that when the work feels too difficult, you can close the book. It will be here for you when you are ready to turn toward your healing once again.

You will meet fellow survivors on your journey through this book. Their stories can bring tears to your eyes as you hold compassion for what they have endured and feel your way into what you also have endured. Holly gives you a front row seat to her work with these survivors, and with it, a chance to take from these illuminating conversations what you also need for yourself.

As Holly reminds you, "Your body has held on to so much." It has. But your body does not need to continue holding on to so much. You get to shed the shame, fear, and pain, so you can create space inside of you for safety, pleasure, and connection. Throughout the book, you will be invited to remind yourself, *"That was then. This is now."* Although your *then* was painful, I am hopeful for all the possibilities that await in your *now*.

Thank you for picking up this book. You are reclaiming control, pleasure, and connection within your life, but the rest of us are also beneficiaries. The less energy you need to expend containing pain and carrying blame, the more energy you have available to share your light, your gifts, and your kindness with the world. Your healing is our healing. Thank you.

—Alexandra H. Solomon, PhD
Author of *Loving Bravely* and
Taking Sexy Back

Healing to Thrive

*It may be that when we no longer know what to do, we have come
to our real work, and that when we no longer know which way to go,
we have come to our real journey.*

—Wendell Berry, *Standing by Words*

I believe you. That's not the problem. The problem is *you* don't believe
you. Or, more accurately, there's a part of you that knows the truth. But
perhaps there's a bigger part that dismisses it, or, at the very least, minimizes it. You are acutely attuned to the inner voice that insists, "It wasn't
that bad. Get over it," followed by the unforgiving question you really
need answered, "Why can't I just move on?"

I know you've tried. Actually, you've done really well. You've buried
your pain and shame at work, school, relationships, and your body. Your
superpower is adornment—putting a high-gloss finish on the exterior
and smiling while your innermost self feels scarred and secretive. You've
given "just moving on" a hell of a go. But eventually, the pain in your
body, the disconnect from people you love, your aversion to sex, or your
insatiable need for it keeps showing up in a way you can't. This has to
change for you to feel fully *you*.

It seems unfair that your accomplishments and tenacity never outshine your mistakes and imperfections (some perceived, some real—
you're human, after all!). You can't get past the failed relationships, lost

friendships, missed promotions, binges, unsuccessful diets, hangovers, and especially that one big mistake. You tune in to that voice again: "I should have said no. I should have known better. It's my fault."

But is it? Is it your fault or is it someone else's? Do you include society in that blame, for not teaching you to use your voice and then not believing you when you do?

This book is for you. I want to affirm your experience, because I know it in my own way. I wanted to write a book to help you wrap your head and heart around what happened—the ways your body took care of you that you mistook for betrayal, and the ways your mind has adapted to the awfulness of what was rather than the goodness of what is.

What if the worst is over?

If you are reading this book, I can almost promise it is. Surviving is the beginning, but not an acceptable end. Are you ready to truly thrive? That is what this book prepares you for: your exquisitely revised story of what comes next. Repairing what you lost to sexual trauma is necessary, even vital to your recovery, *and* it's not enough. I wrote this book to offer you a guide that picks up where most sexual trauma recovery books leave off.

Here's my promise to you: You can renavigate sex and reimagine what is possible for your relational life. In almost every interaction I have with survivors, I see them struggle to feel good about having sex, let alone feel good while having it. Like them, you probably feel broken and unfixable in both wanting and being wanted. I can't tell you how many times I have heard, "Forget it. I don't care if I ever have sex again." But no one can forget it. You do care. You don't need fixing, because *you aren't broken.* You need nurturing and a nudge toward hope.

I have been supporting survivors and watching them reengage with the idea of wanting, of desire, for many years. The recovery of sexual health after sexual assault was the subject of my dissertation and has become the central focus of my work. But the aspiration to put what transpired in a clinical realm—the thoughts and feelings that only existed in the private space between my clients and myself—into a book arose from a concept the esteemed therapist and writer Esther Perel calls "Eros Resurrected."[1]

Perel's concept encouraged me to consider sexual recovery in connection with the power of eroticism. In essence, this is reclamation joining forces with desire. When most people think of "erotic," they probably associate the term with something sexy. But the word "Eros," in the psychological and theoretical sense, means "instinct" or "life force." With this in mind, consider that your journey isn't just about having better sex after trauma but also about creating a more passionate life.

Cultivating Eros includes accessing your innate vibrancy, motivation, creativity, and imagination, and lives entirely in opposition to hopelessness. Eros is belief in your potential and the willingness to demand more. One of my favorite questions to ask is, "Do you want to bet on probability or possibility?" If you remain constricted and guarded, you'll survive. If you step, stretch, and *want*, you'll thrive. Probability is your survivorship. Possibility is your Eros.

Within these pages, I will help you reclaim the sexual and sensual pieces of yourself that you've lost, and also resurrect a drive and appetite for all of the delight, gratification, affection, and intimacy life has to offer you.

After spending more than fourteen thousand hours working with survivors, I know that no matter how exciting this sounds, the process of evolution is scary. It is easier to stay stuck in the mediocre than change for the better. If you think you waited too long to look for help, you haven't. The average length of time it takes a survivor to find their way to my office is ten years, but I've treated survivors as many as fifty years after their trauma. There's no such thing as taking too long to reclaim pleasure, passion, and the life you deserve.

This book is your constant companion and guide. You can jump ahead or go back and reread it again and again, and you may "get" something in your head before you feel it in your body. You probably know the reasons why you are anxious or sad or mad, but don't know how to untether yourself and move forward. Your evolution relies almost exclusively on "how" questions rather than "why" questions. "Why" keeps us stuck in our heads. "How" encourages a process that lets us lean on our bodies, our symptoms, and the way we made it from where we were to where we are.

This "how" is a basic premise of somatic psychology. Reaching understanding through your mind *and* body is called "integration," which is really just a clinical and somewhat elaborate way of saying, "Don't try, just be." Getting over your sexual trauma isn't the goal; getting through it with self-compassion and resilience is.

As you reclaim pleasure and step into thriving, you will replace judgment with acceptance and have a firmer grasp on what you've gained rather than what you've lost. You are here and ready and stronger than you think. I cannot say it any better than author Glennon Doyle at this moment: "I see your pain, and it's big. But I also see your courage, and it's bigger. You can do hard things."[2] You've got this.

Throughout the pages of this book, you will learn it is finally safe to be present. Now is the time to let what you know settle into what you feel. Integration is a core piece of your process, so in that way, this book is designed to help you feel more than it is to help you think. When you get out of your head and into your body, a whole new world of insight and tenderness opens up. My hope is that you can trust what you're feeling.

Because sexual trauma causes psychological, physiological, relational, and sexual harm, we can't fix just one part of this whole-life equation. This book addresses what's happening in our minds and in our bodies, and offers open, honest talk about sex without embarrassment or shame. Reclaiming your sexual health is an indispensable part of your journey, and having good sex necessarily includes consent and pleasure. Feeling safe is a prerequisite for feeling pleasure, but it is only half of the equation for enjoying your best sex and healthiest relationships yet. Thriving is about learning to feel safe and in control, but also enlivened and unbound.

To ground our journey together in safety and trust, here's a brief look ahead. Remember, you always have an exit or the ability to press pause for a while—just close the book when you need to.

Reclaiming Pleasure begins by offering theory and research to help you understand your experience. It presents and explores various types of sexual trauma, what it means to be sexually healthy, what role your body plays, and how to begin to reconcile the ways in which you've survived. Chapters 1 through 5 take a deep dive into dismantling shame. We'll explore using neuroscience and psychophysiology to encourage self-compassion and empathy, and begin the process of separating the suffering of the past from the possibilities of the future. You will read the first of thirteen stories intended to help you recognize yourself through the experiences of other survivors, and to hopefully find motivation in their breakthroughs.

Chapter 6 presents the most common effects of sexual trauma and is designed to help you recognize and gain control of your emotional, physical, sexual, and relational symptoms. These chapters lean heavily on somatic psychology principles that explore the relationship of the body with the mind. Through this exploration, you'll start to bridge the disconnection between the emotional pain you experience in your mind and the physical pain you feel in your body. You'll understand how many of your relational and sexual responses to people and situations were useful *then* but may be problematic *now*—in other words, your symptoms were not behavioral choices, but rather adaptive responses. Your emotions, other people, and—mostly—your body will become forces to return home to rather than run from.

From here, you'll be well prepared for "the work" in chapters 7 through 9, where you'll integrate each facet of your healing. You'll be presented with my three-step process of control, pleasure, and connection, which includes concepts and exercises to help you recognize your blocks and bring awareness to your process of change. Utilizing these distinct elements of recovery, you'll experiment with your perceived limitations and learn to set healthy boundaries, discover how to trust your body's emotional and physical cues, and feel true to yourself and safe in your relationships. You'll also explore *tantra*, which in its ancient Sanskrit translation means "the weave," and focuses on profound connection, not complicated sexual positions (its often-erroneous contemporary interpretation).[3] These chapters will awaken your awareness of what has been lacking, what you have, and what you need to believe differently, feel differently, live differently—and ways you can love differently.

The final chapter looks to the future, offering strategies for translating what happens in the bedroom to the larger scope of your life. You'll be introduced to mindful eroticism through fantasy as a way of deepening the meaning of sex, so it becomes more about presence and less about physicality. This chapter encourages your process of reclamation on an individual level, within your local community as well as the greater global community.

Last but certainly not least, the conclusion is designed to inspire a paradigm shift that not only demands more than surviving after sexual trauma, but in a larger sense, informs strategies for prevention.

When it comes to understanding sexual trauma, it would be an enormous oversight not to highlight the fact that transgender, gender-nonconforming, and nonbinary individuals experience sexual abuse, sexual assault, rape, sexual harassment, and sexual violence at higher percentages than cisgender (non-transgender) people. A 2012 report from the U.S. Department of Justice Office for Victims of Crimes reported transgender people experience sexual assault and sexual abuse at "shockingly higher levels"—up to 66 percent higher—than people outside the trans community.[4] So, while this book is intended for all survivors of sexual trauma and will hopefully be helpful to people of every gender identity, I believe it is essential to offer more targeted resources to anyone reading this who is trans, nonbinary, or gender nonconforming. With that in mind, I recommend *Written on the Body: Letters from Trans and Non-Binary Survivors of Sexual Assault & Domestic Violence*, edited by Lexie Bean, and *Queering Sexual Violence: Radical Voices from within the Anti-Violence Movement*, edited by Jennifer Patterson. These are both thoughtful and thorough references for understanding sexual trauma through a trans and nonbinary lens. I hope that these books might help you fully attend to your unique experience.

This journey you are on to untangle your story, respect your emotions, express your feelings, and return to your body holds at its conclusion the promise of reclamation. Pleasure, Eros, and your ability to thrive are actions experienced in the world, through connection. It is less about doing and more about being. You will prepare, practice, and polish here within these pages, but you will *be* out there, in life and in love.

Your commitment to move beyond surviving is recognized and applauded, and in no way are you alone in this. Thank you for your courage to read this book. That, in and of itself, is a triumph. Please don't get discouraged with your progress, though. You will likely dart ahead and have a string of fantastic days, but then drift back and convince yourself you've gained nothing. One of the things I appreciate most about somatic psychology, and its ultimate goal of cultivating mind-body awareness, is that you can't undo it. You can't un-aware awareness. Once you have it, you have it. However, your newfound tools do require attention and intention in order to work. Keep practicing.

The more you are able to identify with what can be rather than what has been, the easier it will be to embrace the journey of discovery ahead of you. You are on this path to resurrect the connected, empowered, and sexually inspired life you deserve.

Traveler, there is no path.
The path is made by walking.

—Antonio Machado

CHAPTER ONE

Understanding Your Trauma

The most fundamental aggression to ourselves, the most fundamental harm we can do to ourselves, is to remain ignorant by not having the courage and respect to look at ourselves honestly and gently.

—Pema Chödrön, *When Things Fall Apart*

Sexuality is an experience of connection. It is how we express ourselves erotically—to others and ourselves—that lets us know our uniqueness is felt emotionally and physically. Sexual trauma dramatically reduces our range of expression, leaving us with fewer words, less tolerable access to touch, and more tenuous relational bonds.

Before we begin, I will suggest that you have a journal that you keep handy for this work. It's essential in many of the exercises and will help you track your journey. It doesn't need to be anything fancy. Just make sure you have it nearby as we progress.

Throughout this book, I share other people's stories because they offer gateways to your own expansion; the unfurling of *more* that you have been tentatively searching for but haven't dared to fully want. It is other people's stories, which we would never judge as harshly as our own, that can crack open our protective shell. Cracks are how the light gets in, after all. It's my hope that you won't use more bandages to cover them, but instead, you'll take the opportunity to let light shine through them.

With your burgeoning sexual self in mind, I offer this first story as you set off to thrive.

Story: *Throwing the Curtains Back*

My first session with Shanna starts as many sessions do, with an exchange of niceties and paperwork followed by a few terrifying seconds when she realizes what she's done: she has come to tell a complete stranger her biggest secret. I read her face and body language—her eyes are wide and she barely blinks as she scooches back on the couch, as far away from me as she can get. I let her know that today's session will be about getting to know each other, and we most likely wouldn't go into anything too difficult. She relaxes a bit and we begin talking, but she quickly stops herself mid-sentence and says, "I feel like I have to tell you. Can I tell you?"

Shanna, like many, has kept her secret for too long. She is hurting and desperate for help, and is sure if she walks out of this office still holding her most painful truth, she'll never come back. She feels brave today but is unwilling to bet on herself tomorrow. She knows if she doesn't get her story out right this minute, she'll have to swallow it one more time, and this time she's sure she'll choke. Without having the fully formed thought in her head, she somehow understands that telling leads to healing. Shame prospers in the shadow of secrets, but Shanna's about to throw the curtains back.

Shanna sits on her hands and tells her story to my bookshelf, avoiding eye contact. I understand. She's ready to speak but not ready to be seen. I take her cue and look at my notepad. "I was sexually assaulted, I'm pretty sure, by a guy in college. I know he did stuff to me because I had a lot of pain there," she says looking down at her lap. "But I don't remember all of it because I was drinking. I mean, I must have passed out. I think I said something, but maybe I didn't. I remember leaving the bar with him."

And then she looks at me. In a voice stronger than I've heard so far, she says, "I'm too scared to even go on a date and it's been, like, eight years. I don't get it. What's wrong with me?"

This is the part Shanna needs me to hear. She is convincing and absolute in her frustration and self-blame, much less so in the truth of her suffering. And she's right—she doesn't get it. If she is going to change how she feels, she has to explore what she knows, or more accurately, what she believes. We will go slowly and start dismantling the narrative she's accepted: the one where she's the antagonist and problem-causer rather than the protagonist and problem-solver, whistleblower, supporter, and redeemer. As much as I know this is a long and deliberate process, I want her to have a glimpse of how her story unfolds.

I answer her question, which, like most survivors, was more of a statement than a query, and say, "There's nothing wrong with you."

She hasn't broken our gaze. She wants to believe me and is assessing every possible cue to see if I'm intentionally misleading her or possibly placating her just to be nice. I repeat, "There's nothing wrong with you," and add, "Something happened to you. That's different."

Shanna shifts positions again and I know we are done discussing the past for today. We come back to the present and talk about her successes since her trauma. After some prompting, she shares a few areas of her present life that she's proud of. In our last few minutes, I decide to take a step into the future and ask, "What do you want for yourself?"

There is a long pause. Most survivors know they aren't happy with what is, but they haven't dared to dream about what could be.

"I don't want to be scared anymore," she replies quietly.

I accept her answer, but press for more: "You will feel less scared. I'm sure of that. But what's beyond not being scared? What's the next thing you want?"

She looks down at her lap again, trying to access one small part of herself that believes she can do more than exist. She finally looks up, shrugs her shoulders, and says, "I want to know what I want. I only know what I don't want."

I tell her most survivors need to embrace the power of "no" before they have their yeses, and that the way she's doing it, by leading with "no," has been a smart and safe way to move through the world. And then I say, "In this moment, you're exactly where you should be. Thank you for letting me know where you want to go."

Story Reflections

In your journal, reflect on how you relate to Shanna's story.

Do you notice yourself feeling sad or angry about what happened to Shanna, or excited and hopeful for her as she begins to heal? Or even both?

What feeling best describes how you feel about your own journey of recovery?

What scares you most about your journey?

What excites you most about it?

Cultivating Clarity

We can't start with what we don't know! To begin healing from sexual trauma, it is essential that we understand it, that we are all on common ground. Words like "rape," "assault," "abuse," and "harassment" are often used interchangeably, and while there are common threads connecting these terms, they are all different experiences. Providing clarity around the specifics of sexual trauma will help ground you in fact, not conjecture. And, in a subtler way, these words let you know you are not alone—if your experience is here in a book, on a page, it is real and hasn't only happened to you. Sexual trauma in particular is a wound that expands in isolation. Shame settles into secrets, and sometimes it takes bringing the hidden parts of yourself to the foreground to feel the collective embrace of others who have similarly suffered. Only when you are aware of what happened, without self-judgment and blame, can you accept it, recover from it, and move past it.

Shanna's story reinforces the need for accurate language to acknowledge sexual trauma in a discerning way. Sometimes you may use an inexact word because it is self-protective: "She touched me" rather than "She sexually abused me," or "He assaulted me" rather than "He raped me." True, it sounds less violent and less severe to say someone touched you rather than abused you. But then, imagine what might happen when your new, kind, and thoughtful partner says, "I'd love to touch you." How do you hold your two opposing realities of the word "touch"? Touch is not malevolent; assault is.

Other times, you may simply not know which words accurately describe your trauma. In our first session, Shanna said "sexual assault" instead of "rape," the latter of which was more accurate. I guessed this by her description of her pain and injuries, and she confirmed during our second session that her perpetrator penetrated her. Having accurate terminology for her trauma did not make her journey any harder—or any less hard—just more balanced and less self-critical because she could connect the intensity of her feelings to the magnitude of her truth.

The way we communicate is critical to recovery because *words inform our experience.*[5] If we hear or say something enough (even in our heads), we start to believe it.

One of the foundations of your shift toward pleasure and passion is exploring how you see yourself. Specifically, do you identify as a survivor of sexual trauma or as a victim of sexual trauma? Notice the difference in tone, spirit, and resonance of the word "survivor" versus "victim." If you and I were sitting together for a therapy session and I continually referred to you as a victim of sexual trauma, you might eventually internalize this message and your experience could be one of continued distress and disempowerment. If I call you a survivor of sexual trauma, you are more likely to identify with your strengths and have an experience of perseverance and empowerment.

Of course, there can be power in identifying as a victim, too, if you feel that most accurately describes where you are in your healing journey. I do want to meet you where you are. But because "survivor" is such a powerful way of naming the reality of what you are, that's the term this book will use (with the exception of our discussion of the "victim mindset," about disengaging from a particular, pernicious belief system, in chapter 5). And either way, I urge you to explore what labels you use to describe yourself and your experience with sexual trauma, and what this says about where you are right now.

Language Reflections

In your journal, write down your answers to these questions.

How do you feel when you say, out loud, the word "victim"?

How do you feel when you say, out loud, the word "survivor"?

Have you identified as either in the past?

How does it feel to identify as a survivor? ("Scary" or "I'm not sure I'm ready" are perfectly fine answers. Your place at these beginning moments may simply be with one toe in the water of hope. It is a good start!)

Like Shanna, most people lack knowledge about different types of sexual trauma. It may be that we don't know because we don't want to know, which is understandable but not practical, unfortunately. Even mental and sexual health professionals are often confused, namely from a lack of comprehensive training. Words offer us a first step forward, providing clarity where it has been lacking and helping you find your foundation in information rather than supposition. The following terms are not exhaustive by any means, but do offer an overview of the most common types of sexual trauma and frequently used terms.

If one or two resonate deeply, particularly if you have not had the insight before, I encourage you to do more research (check out "Your Allies and Resources Guide" at the end of this book). This is your chance to merge the awareness of what you thought about your trauma with what you now know about it.

Clarifying Terms

Consent is the act of communicating agreement to participate in sexual activity at the time the sexual activity is occurring. This can be communicated through words or actions—including body language—and must be given freely. If the agreement is in any way forced through pressure, manipulation, or coercion, it is considered nonconsensual because permission was not given voluntarily.[6]

Rape is the term used for sexual intercourse, penetration, or oral sex, with or without force, without consent. The most recent legal definition of rape is, "Unlawful sexual activity that includes penetration, no matter how slight, of the vagina or anus with any body part or object, or oral penetration by a sex organ of another person, without the consent of the survivor."[7] Rape is a form of sexual assault, but not all sexual assault is rape.[8]

Rape can happen to people of all ages, genders, sexual orientations, ethnicities, geographical locations, cultures, economic circumstances, and degrees of physical or psychological impairment. There are different subsets of rape, which include sodomy, date rape, gang rape, marital or spousal rape, acquaintance rape, and stranger rape. Acquaintance rape and date rape, in which the survivor knows the perpetrator to some degree, are the most common. Because most survivors know their perpetrator, rape is significantly underreported. Rape can be committed over a long period of time with little to no physical injury. Consent and penetration are the only two determining factors of rape, not violence or force. In the United States, one in every six women and one in every seventy-one men will experience rape in their lifetime. Ninety percent of rape survivors are women and 10 percent are male.[9]

Rape culture is a sociological concept for a setting in which sexual violence is both prevalent and normalized due to pervasive attitudes about sex and gender. Common attributes of rape culture thinking include slut shaming, survivor blaming, sexual objectification, trivializing, and denying all types of sexual violence and sexual harassment.[10]

Sexual abuse, also referred to as *molestation,* is the perpetration of any type of sexual behavior toward a person who is unable to give consent because of age (a minor), physical inability, or developmental disability.[11] Types of sexual abuse include touch, penetration, indecent exposure, coercion, sexual exploitation (sex trafficking), exposure to pornography, or forced participation in pornography. Sexual abuse by a family member is considered incest. Globally, 18 to 19 percent of women and 8 percent of men report being sexually abused[12] and 93 percent of sexual abuse survivors know their perpetrators.[13]

The differences in criteria across U.S. state laws, for instance, can make it hard for some people to understand their sexual abuse *as* abuse. My clinical rule of thumb, particularly if a survivor is struggling to remember their exact age or their perpetrator's age when the abuse happened, is this: if it felt abusive, it was abusive.

Sexual abuse can be difficult, if not impossible, for survivors to recognize when it first begins because it often doesn't feel wrong. Most sexual abuse, especially when perpetrated by a family member or family friend, starts with extra attention, additional caretaking, gifts, and special outings. It often isn't until survivors are older and have more social and cognitive awareness (unless pain was being inflicted) that they understand what happened was wrong and illegal. Sexual abuse does not have to be forceful; it only needs to be nonconsensual. Minors or people with disabilities can never consent when there is an age or power disparity.

Sexual assault includes a wide range of unwanted acts that are sexual in nature and occur without consent, up to but not including penetration of or with the genitals. They can either be completed or attempted against the survivor's will or when consent cannot be given due to a physical or mental condition, including the influence of alcohol or drugs. Sexual assault may involve actual or threatened physical force, use of weapons, coercion, or intimidation. It can include attempted rape, unwanted touching or fondling, close proximity and unwanted exposure to a person masturbating, forced oral sex, or penetration of the perpetrator's body. Sexual assault can also include acts of online aggression where the perpetrator exposes themself.

Sexual assault is often used as a comprehensive term to describe any nonconsensual sexual behavior perpetrated against an adult. Sexual assault is the largest and broadest category of reported sex crimes, occurring globally with presence in all social, economic, ethnic, racial, religious, and age groups.[14] Sexual assault happens to men, women, and nonbinary individuals, though the prevalence of perpetration against women is highest, at least in incidents that are reported. A 2013 study by the National Crime Victimization Survey found 89.3 percent of survivors of sexual assault are women, while 10.7 percent are men.[15] The Rape, Abuse & Incest National Network (RAINN) reports that every 73 seconds, a person in the United States is sexually assaulted.[16] Global estimates published by the World Health Organization (WHO) in 2017 indicated that one in three (35 percent) of women worldwide have experienced sexual assault in their lifetime.[17]

Sexual assault can be difficult to recognize because the perpetrator is almost always an acquaintance of the survivor. In fact, eight out of ten sexual assaults are committed by someone known to the survivor; 33 percent of perpetrators are former or current partners or spouses.[18] This makes the emotional transgression particularly hard for survivors to discern, and legal confrontation that much more arduous. A survivor may believe that because they had consensual sex at a certain time(s) with their perpetrator, they will not be believed about a specific transgression. Sharing and promoting the fact that most sexual assaults are perpetrated by someone the survivor knows may help diminish the shame and offer increased opportunities for support.

Sexual harassment is behavior characterized by coercion, unwanted attention, inappropriate sexual remarks, or physical advances in professional or social situations. There is almost always a power disparity, through which the perpetrator feels empowered and the survivor feels disempowered. A 2018 survey by the nonprofit organization Stop Street Harassment, analyzed by the Center for Gender Equality and Health, found 81 percent of women and 43 percent of men had experienced some form of sexual harassment during their lifetime.[19]

Offensive physical touch often does not happen in cases of harassment, but words and gestures are used to humiliate and create fear. This fear can stem from a perceived likelihood of bodily harm, a jeopardized career, lost earning potential, disclosure of personal information, or name-calling (catcalling or slut-shaming). The cases surrounding the #MeToo movement are contemporary examples of ways sexual harassment occurs.[20] It is often subtle and manipulative on the part of the perpetrator—they may even use humor or flirtation—which makes the exchange confusing for the survivor.

Gender harassment is a subset of sexual harassment, and more specifically describes harassment that occurs because of someone's gender identity.

Sexual offender refers to someone who perpetrated a nonconsensual sexual act and has been convicted of a criminal sexual offense.

Sexual perpetrator refers to a person who obtains or tries to obtain sexual contact with another person, regardless of whether they are a minor or an adult, without consent.

Sexual pleasure is the physical and/or psychological satisfaction and enjoyment derived from solitary or shared erotic experiences, including thoughts, dreams, and autoeroticism.[21]

Sexual predator is typically used pejoratively to describe a person who has committed or continually tries to commit multiple sexual offenses, whether they were convicted of those crimes or not.

Sexual trauma is a broad term that refers to one or multiple sexual violations of any kind that invoke significant distress. It is a term used clinically (though generally not legally or empirically) because it allows for a wider gradation of scope and ambiguity in labeling the experience. It also offers survivors, clinicians, and supporters terminology for collectively understanding without stigmatizing, which can happen when details and descriptions are provided in a more exacting way. Using the term "sexual trauma" is an appropriate and accurate way to describe any unwanted sexual experience in a clinical or social setting.

Sexual violence is a broad term that encompasses forcing or manipulating another person into unwanted sexual activity. Sexual violence can happen to anyone at any age and comprises sexual abuse, sexual assault, rape, and sexual harassment. The majority of sexual violence is perpetrated against women, but sexual violence against men is a significant problem, and one that has been largely neglected in research. Global estimates range from 3 to 13 percent, with a large portion of perpetration occurring in prison systems.[22] Sexual violence also incorporates online aggression, including stalking, nonconsensual sharing of photos or videos, sexualized bullying, revenge porn, and gender violence. Like sexual trauma, sexual violence is a comprehensive term that can be used to talk about the offense without being explicit or detailed. Often survivors use the term "sexual violence" rather than "sexual trauma" if their experience felt specifically forceful, whether physically or emotionally.

Survivor is used to describe someone who has experienced any type of sexual trauma. More specifically, it is most often applied to someone who has gone through the recovery process, or when addressing the short- or long-term effects of sexual trauma.[23] It is seen as identifying and unifying language in the sexual violence prevention community.

Victim is typically used when referring to someone who has recently experienced sexual violence or who did not survive a sexually violent attack. It is also used when discussing legal aspects within the criminal justice system.[24] Many practitioners and anti-sexual violence advocates do not use the term "victim" because they believe it has pathologizing consequences.

Clarifying Terms Reflections

Use your journal to reflect on these terms.

How would you prefer to define and communicate about your sexual trauma? (Examples: "I am a survivor of sexual abuse." "I experienced sexual violence in high school." "Sexual harassment happened to me at my previous job." "I have experienced several sexual traumas.")

How are you replacing assumption and judgment about your sexual trauma with understanding and compassion?

Is there anything you feel now about your sexual trauma that you have not felt before?

You Are Not Your Trauma

Being able to name what happened to you will help create stability within you. You will begin to feel a separation between your *self* and your *experience*. You are not your trauma. Many people have never considered themselves survivors because they didn't think their trauma was "bad" enough. This first chapter is an offering of awareness: I want you to know that what happened to you was categorically wrong and sufficiently bad. And you survived. As a reminder, sexual transgressions of any nature do not need to be violent; they only need to be nonconsensual. If you did not say yes, consent was not given. I cannot tell you how many times I have spoken these words: "I don't care if you were sitting on a street corner naked. Most people would have brought you a coat. The only reason you were raped is because a rapist walked by."

This line of thinking is true for other types of sexual trauma as well. You were abused because of an abuser; you were assaulted because of a perpetrator; you were harassed because of a sexual predator. Here and now is your first step toward placing blame solidly where it belongs—on someone other than yourself.

Blame Reflections

Write these down in your journal. Take your time. These aren't easy questions to answer.

What aspects of your sexual trauma did you believe were your fault?

Where should blame for your sexual trauma be placed?

In what ways are you not responsible for what happened?

If you have not told your story to another person—if you have never spoken the words out loud—rest assured, it is not necessary in order to completely heal and fully reclaim pleasure. It isn't the details that matter. In fact, some of the most inspiring stories are those in which few details surrounding the trauma are shared.

You were not in control of what happened during your trauma, but you are in control of what happens in your healing. That may mean protecting the discrete facets of your experience, or, like Shanna, exposing the details may feel crucial, prompting a necessary step away from shame. Replacing presumption with information and judgment with compassion allows you to experience the full range of emotions, from heartbroken to courageously determined. With this knowledge, I believe you are ready to take the next steps in healing.

Having a thorough understanding of your sexual trauma and what you've been through offers a necessary foothold on where you're going. Next, we will work on opening the lens beyond trauma to view your assumptions and deep-seated beliefs about sexuality. Rather than seeing your inherent sexuality as something to be feared and protected, the next chapter presents an opportunity for it to be wholly appreciated and respected.

CHAPTER TWO

In Search of Sexual Health

*Sexuality is at the core of human personality; it's not what you do,
but who you are.*

—Patricia Fuller

If there has been one glaring omission in the sexual trauma recovery field, it has been a lack of focus on sexual health. This absence—the gap between where you are and where you deserve to be—is at the core of your process of reclamation. Sexual trauma is incredibly difficult to acknowledge, and when overlaid with negative cultural and familial belief systems about sex in general, prioritizing your sexual health becomes even harder. We live in a society where talking about sexuality is often considered taboo unless it is commercialized, humorized, or catered to the traditional patriarchal gaze. We are spoon-fed "no's" and starved of "yeses." Early on, you most likely received these types of messages: "Don't get pregnant," "Don't get a sexually transmitted infection (STI)," "Don't be promiscuous, but don't be a prude." But I bet you never heard a word about the naturalness of your libido! Were you ever told that you could trust it rather than fear it, or taught to ask for what you want or what feels good? Most of us never were.

If you were raised to believe sex is inherently bad, dirty, or shameful, becoming sexually healthy may feel like an untenable paradox to manage. When you externalize sex as something you *do* (like a job), rather than an internal and essential part of your well-being (like your heartbeat), you cut off something you can't live without. If you can't talk about sex— the gifts it can offer, not just the scars it has left—you can't talk about living your most healthy, fulfilling, and empowered life. Sexual health isn't a bonus; it's a necessity.

Your ability to be your most healthy sexual self includes factors like culture, age, religion, family, education, and socioeconomic status. Similar to your exploration of sexual trauma in chapter 1, it is equally important to deepen your understanding of sexual health. One lives in juxtaposition to the other, and it's the gap in between that must be tended to. In Emily Nagoski's groundbreaking book on the science of sex, *Come as You Are*, she writes, "When a person experiences trauma, it's like someone snuck into their garden and ripped out all of the plants they had been cultivating with such care and attention...There is rage and betrayal, there is grief for the garden as it was, and there is fear that it will never grow back."[25]

Reclaiming your sexual health, including what you were born with, what you were and weren't given, and what you lost, is the replanting of *your* garden. There is no part of your sexually healthy self that can evolve in shadows. Given enough thoughtfulness and light, you will grow.

Story: *Queen of Getting the Guy*

Manali had been sexually abused by her uncle during her preteen years and now, at twenty-eight, was struggling to have a sexually healthy relationship. She excelled at work, made friends easily, and had a dry sense of humor that was instantly endearing. "I'm queen of getting the guy, but I quickly become Cinderella and 'poof,' my prince is gone," she explained, with a dramatic flick of her fingers and an eye roll.

Our first two months of sessions were dedicated to understanding her trauma and rewriting her story, one in which she became her own savior rather than a victim of an incestuous pedophile. Manali was clever, and even at age thirteen, she figured out a way to make her uncle stop by threatening to reveal the horrible secret to her father, his brother. She admitted that she still isn't certain she could have followed through, but luckily, he was unwilling to call her bluff and the abuse stopped. Manali went on to graduate high school and college with honors, and secured a great job. By focusing on doing rather than feeling, she thought she was safe and the pain was behind her. Her step through the door of the rape crisis center where we met was a huge acknowledgment that her past hadn't stopped sabotaging her present. "I always get left because of sex," she stated. "In the beginning I feel adored, sometimes even loved. But I've had more than one boyfriend tell me I'm like sleeping with a dead fish."

Manali had partners stay for as long as ten months, hanging in there because they thought sex would get better, but most of her relationships lasted less than two months. She was frustrated that all her successes and smarts weren't providing an answer. She had "fixed" everything else in her life after the sexual abuse, so she wondered why sex and relationships weren't falling in line too.

"What are your expectations about sex?" I asked.

For the first time there was no witty comeback. Manali had been serious and thoughtful when considering her childhood trauma, but when she talked about herself as an adult, she lacked sensitivity and her responses were couched in sarcasm. There was little room to feel how painful her present circumstance—loneliness and hopelessness—was.

"What do I expect?" she asked. "Umm, I guess that he, uh, finishes," though her response was more of a question than an answer.

"What do you expect for you?" I pushed. "What do you want to feel?"

Manali was quiet, her face blank as if I suddenly started speaking another language. It turns out I had. I was asking her to think about physical intimacy and her own eroticism, which was a foreign subject from an unheard-of land. "I'm lost," she finally said through tears.

"You're not. You've just never been shown a map," I said. "Maybe a better analogy is that I'm handing you a menu of foods you've never tasted and asking you to tell me what you like. You won't know until you try."

Manali had never explored her body as a source of pleasure, had never masturbated, had never looked at her own genitals, had never said the words "orgasm" or "come," had never asked her partner what they liked, and had certainly never considered what she liked. There was no sex education in her high school, and she had never discussed anything sexual with her parents or friends. Over the next several months she was able to keep the past in the past and recognize the role her trauma played in suppressing her sexual health versus the role her upbringing and complete lack of sex education played. "I'm bad at sex not because I'm scared anymore, but because I have no idea how to do it. I expect to be told what to do. I don't know if I'm more embarrassed or mad at myself," she stated.

In pure Manali style, her frustration led to hard work and a deep dive into exploring her body, sensuality, sexuality, and pleasure. She took a six-month break from dating apps to devote time to taking herself on dates. This included solo dinners at nice restaurants, lots of sci-fi movies at her favorite arthouse theater, belly dancing lessons, and the purchase of three vibrators. She wanted to ensure the improvement of her sexual health was on as solid ground as her sexual trauma recovery.

During our last session, we discussed what she had lost, gained, and still hoped to achieve. Manali said, "My sexual abuse took so much from me. I never got the exciting first kiss or sexual experience that most people do. My uncle stole that. But it's just as sad that I never got a fair shot at being sexually healthy, even if the trauma hadn't happened. I'm doing it differently this time. It's a second chance I never expected, but one that I am so grateful for."

Story Reflections

Manali's struggles with reclaiming sexual health were present because of her sexual abuse, but also because she never had any type of education or open communication about sexuality. Sexual trauma is a part of your story that is holding you back from being your most healthy sexual self, but it is often not the whole story. Don't give your trauma more power than it deserves. In your journal, reflect on how you relate to Manali's story.

How was sex spoken about in your home?

From whom or what did you learn about sex? Was it from school, friends, magazines, rom-coms, pornography, or some other source?

What words in regard to body parts or sexual acts are you uncomfortable saying out loud? Practice in private!

What roadblocks to being sexually healthy has your trauma triggered?

What roadblocks to being sexually healthy has your upbringing evoked?

An Inside Job

Like Manali, you have your own innate resiliencies and impediments. What does being sexually healthy mean to you? First and foremost, particularly from a mind-body approach, it's about embracing the idea that your sexuality is as unique to you as your eye color, hair color, skin tone, and personality traits. In *Phenomenology of Perception*, Maurice Merleau-Ponty conceptualized the nondual foundation of sexuality and self, establishing that one cannot exist without the other.[26] This means that if you don't own your sexuality, you can't fully own your *self*. When you work to restore your sexual health, or perhaps construct it for the first time, you step into a way of thinking (mind) and a way of feeling (body) that you and you alone are in control of—not your perpetrator, not your family, not the culture you were raised in, not what was forced on you, not what was disregarded.

Sexual health is an inside job that includes your brain, your heart, and all of your erogenous, feel-so-good zones. From this moment forward, you have the choice to unpack and affirm all facets of your sexuality, and those choices fundamentally encompass your entire sense of well-being. And while your sexual identity isn't a choice, openly affirming that you are bisexual, gay, or queer often is. (Stepping out of the closet is hard!) Even if "asexual" is how you sexually identify, it is a recognition *about* your sexuality, not an omission of it. Similarly, when made from a foundation of sexual health, being nonmonogamous, figuring out you like kissing but dislike oral sex, or that sexting turns you on but porn does not, are all choices based on innate personal preferences, not beliefs or judgments.

Reading definitions may not be the most exciting part of your journey, but as you discovered in chapter 1, truly understanding what we are talking about must precede our assumptions. "Sexual trauma" and "sexual health" are terms offered frequently with the supposition of discernment, while in reality few of us have ever taken a moment to ask, "What do they mean?"

Coming to an agreed-upon definition of sexual health has not been without struggle, even for those committed to improving it, most notably in the domains of research and public policy. An attempt at universal consensus began in 1975 when the World Health Organization (WHO) expanded the focus of sexual health beyond unwanted pregnancy and absence of disease: "Sexual health is the integration of somatic, emotional, intellectual, and social aspects of sexual being, in ways that are positively enriching and that enhance personality, communication, and love."[27]

It was a contemplative but somewhat abstract start for an essential part of our well-being that, at its core, is supposed to be safe and feel good! Over two decades later, WHO teamed up with the World Association for Sexual Health (WAS) to create a definition that finally spoke to safety and pleasure, two critical elements of your ability to live healthfully and passionately:

> *Sexual health is a state of physical, emotional, mental, and social well-being related to sexuality; it is not merely the absence of disease, dysfunction, or infirmity. Sexual health requires a positive and respectful approach to sexuality and sexual relationships, as well as the possibility of having pleasurable and safe sexual experiences, free of coercion, discrimination, and violence. For sexual health to be attained and maintained, the sexual rights of all persons must be respected, protected, and fulfilled.*[28]

Yes! There it is. And it's a mouthful. I often email it to clients and encourage them to write it on a card and place it somewhere easily visible as a daily reminder of what they are entitled to. But when working with survivors on the specifics of their unique version of sexual health, I use a more linear and somewhat easier to digest description. The following list is from venerated sex therapist Douglas Braun-Harvey and stands easily and strikingly in opposition to sexual trauma.[29] The Six Principles of Sexual Health are:

1. Consent

2. Nonexploitation

3. Protection from HIV/STIs and unintended pregnancy

4. Honesty

5. Shared values

6. Mutual pleasure

Sexual health is a multifaceted cornerstone of your overall well-being, and a right to be safeguarded and treasured. Immersing yourself in your unique choices about sexual health instead of familial, cultural, or trauma-informed programming is a foundational step on your journey to pleasure, passion, and loving relationships.

Clarifying Terms Reflections

Use your journal to reflect on these terms.

First, notice how sexual health is entirely at odds with sexual trauma. What surprises you most?

Write the definition of sexual health that resonates most deeply with you on a card or piece of paper (or as your phone background!) and place somewhere easily visible.

Which elements of sexual health have you thought about? Which have you not previously considered?

Other than consent, which principle is most important to you? (You can choose more than one if you want.)

Consider how each principle was revoked or devalued during your trauma.

Consider how you can begin to prioritize and value these principles in the future.

A Sex-Positive Approach

The term "sex positive" is garnering increased attention in everything from women's magazines and relationship podcasts to dissertation topics; however, like the concept of healthy sexuality, many people know sex positivity is a good thing to have but don't truly understand what it means. There are multiple definitions of sex positivity, all of which are valid and add constructive insight to the discourse on human sexuality, but there's one that's stunningly simple, is easy to remember, and exposes the heart of what all sex should be. It has nothing to do with positions, or orgasms, or what your body looks like. It won't minimize what hurt you, and can't normalize something that will never be normal. This definition has the potential to completely reframe your trauma—and obliterate the possibility of additional traumas—by shining a spotlight on two certitudes that refuse to return to the shadows.

The sex-positive definition that I want you to fully embrace is this: *All sex is good sex as long as it's consensual and pleasurable.*

Say this out loud. Now, say it again. Why? Because saying things out loud rather than to yourself is a somatic psychology principle that creates a *lived experience* of a thought or feeling rather than a cognitive experience of it. Simplified, lived experience is defined as "I can do this, not just *think* this." Saying things out loud puts thought in motion and adds actions to your beliefs. So, one more time, say it out loud: *All sex is good sex as long as it's consensual and pleasurable.*

Filtering your sexual experiences—past, present, and future—through a lens of sex positivity leaves no room for confusion about what you deserve. Remember, sexual trauma doesn't have to be violent; it only has to be nonconsensual. Ask yourself, "Was it consensual?" Then ask, "Was it pleasurable?" To make sure you are 100 percent solid on your definitions of consent and pleasure, please take a quick glance back at chapter 1. Consent and pleasure are the centerpiece of your recipe for great, healthy sex! We'll dig deeper into how to prepare these two ingredients (you can add flavor to consent and pleasure in dozens of ways), but there is no good meal without them.

I know you have struggled to figure out what's sexually acceptable, what's "good enough." This is a bottom-of-the-barrel expectation, and has no place in your story of reclamation. Just as it is your right to demand consent, it is also your right to demand pleasure! Saying "meh" after sex? Take that option off the table.

The self-protective warrior in you has minimized your trauma in order to make living and loving tolerable, so questions around what's right, what's wrong, what's good, what's bad, what's a "yes," or what's a "no" have likely become muddled. In addition to your trauma, you may have had other sexual experiences that weren't entirely consensual. They weren't explicitly rape or abuse or assault or harassment, but they may have left you feeling bad about what happened and even worse about yourself. Like most survivors, I'm guessing you barely considered *your* pleasure during sexual experiences, even during those that checked the "consensual" box. The absolute concreteness of sex positivity clears the water, finally. By embracing this concept of sex positivity, your days of ambiguity and tolerance of anything less than gratifying will hopefully be over. Consent and pleasure are the only acceptable footholds from which to rebuild both your relational and your sexual life.

Sex-Positive Reflections

Write down and then repeat it out loud: *All sex is good sex as long as it's consensual and pleasurable.*

How have your beliefs about consent shifted?

How is the concept of consent no longer ambiguous?

How has your perspective on pleasure changed?

Do you believe you deserve pleasure? How do you know—do you feel it somewhere in your body? Where?

In what ways, through your unique version of sexual health, can pleasure begin to be prioritized?

Your process of reclaiming what you deserve rests on pillars of consent and pleasure. You picked up this book because you are a survivor and have committed yourself to ensuring consent is present at every turn. Please dedicate yourself to ensuring pleasure is present too! You'll get specific guidelines on how to put pleasure front and center in chapter 8, but for now, it stands on its own merit as a principle to be pursued. Sexual trauma is entirely at odds with sexual health and a sex-positive belief system. You know what you don't want. Now it's time to discover what you do want.

Can you imagine your body as a reliable friend, not as an untrustworthy enemy? As we look ahead at your process of reclamation, we necessarily turn our focus to your body. The experience of sex at its worst and at its best happens in your body, so your body will become your intuitive launchpad for healing. Chapter 3 presents your first exposure to mind-body exercises, and offers a chance to understand how your body processes trauma and ways in which you can compassionately attend to your past without holding on to it.

Though your body may feel dangerous or even repulsive to you at these early stages, much of your survivor story will be rewritten here. You have already begun to remember your trauma in a way that allows you to think about it differently. Now you'll begin to re-member it, somatically speaking, by putting the pieces back together to settle into your body in an unfamiliar though extraordinary way. This is the time to stop running from your body and instead come home to it. Thought by thought, breath by breath, and bone by bone, your ideal balance of safety and vitality are waiting.

CHAPTER THREE

Minding the Body

When one is pretending, the entire body revolts.

—Anaïs Nin, *Winter of Artifice*

Do you feel like your body "goes without you"? That's how many survivors describe the experience of disconnection between their mind and body during sexual trauma, but also, and perhaps more so, in the months and years that follow. Maybe you're sitting at a restaurant with friends or walking down the street in broad daylight and suddenly feel unsafe. Even if there is no obvious threat, your heart races, your stomach churns, and you can't catch your breath. Or perhaps you're in bed with a trustworthy partner, but out of nowhere your body tenses and their touch feels repulsive. In both of these instances you become confused and exasperated because everything seems all right, yet your body is screaming, "No it's not!" So how is this happening? This kind of situation is a continuation of the story you've been telling yourself. You likely perceive this type of reaction as a flaw on your part for what you can't do, rather than a huge failing on your perpetrator's part for what they did.

When we look at sexual trauma solely through a cognitive lens (meaning we try to understand and move through only what we know, not what we feel), we miss a huge part of the recovery equation. Since sexual trauma happens in the body, it must be healed through the body. What you're feeling in those seemingly inexplicable and frustrating moments is what I call your Survivor Security System (SSS) in action, which is both a lifesaver and sometimes slightly—or significantly—overzealous, like a well-intentioned best friend. Your SSS speaks in a language your body understands but your mind has trouble translating. The goal, once again, is integration, which lands your body and mind on the same page. As trauma therapist Bessel van Der Kolk writes, "You can be fully in charge of your life only if you can acknowledge the reality of your body, in all its visceral dimensions."[30]

Story: *I've Been Here Before*

"It's coming back," Alex said through a cracked voice. "I've barely thought about it for three years, but I felt it and it's coming back."

Alex was afraid he didn't have control of his secret and it was wielding its ugly head, ready to bite him when he wasn't looking. Like many survivors, he knew he had been sexually assaulted but put the memory of his trauma in a locked box and buried it. He'd have flashbacks to that night every now and then but could quickly capture the thought and shove it back in the box. Compartmentalization—the ability to subconsciously defend against conflicting feelings—hadn't just become a common practice for Alex, but a perfected art form. "It was like it happened to another person, still me but a different me," he tried to explain.

"How do you know it's coming back?" I asked.

I didn't need to know the specifics of what was coming back or details of his trauma. I only needed to know how he was so sure his past was invading his present. Without missing a beat, he answered, "Because the hair on the back of my neck stood up."

"Wow, there's your body keeping you safe," I replied.

He looked at me with exasperation and said, "But I wasn't in danger. I was just trying to go for a run."

I told him that sometimes our bodies have access to feelings our minds don't, and explained, "This is actually a good sign. It means the process of integration is happening, which is when your mind and body make a pact that it's time to heal."

Alex took a deep breath and started to tell me what he remembered, apologizing frequently for what he didn't. "You don't need to remember every detail," I offered. "Just stick with what you feel. Your body is already doing that for you. Trust it. You're safe now."

Alex recounted a night at a club in Manhattan, on the Lower East Side. He drank champagne and flirted with several guys, eventually ending up in a group with a private room and bottle service. "My glass just kept getting refilled, but I don't feel like I drank that much. It's hard for me to believe I blacked out on champagne, but I can't figure out what happened."

The next morning, he woke up in an unfamiliar apartment to a man stroking his penis and kissing him. He remembers sitting up quickly and the man stopping. "Then he asked me if I wanted toast," Alex recalled. "I said yes."

At this point Alex curled up in a tight ball on my couch and cried. After several minutes he looked up and asked, "What is wrong with me? Why was I nice? Why did I eat toast with this creepy jerk? It's disgusting."

By "disgusting" I presumed Alex meant both the assault and his initial reaction to it, more emphasis on the latter. He never told anyone because he thought it was his fault—he drank too much and was nice to the guy. In his mind, those two things couldn't add up to sexual assault. "I got out of the apartment quickly after the toast and took a cab home. I knew I was uptown, but barely have any memories of that morning either. I had to be at work at Abercrombie at 4 p.m., so that's what I did. Life just went on as usual after that. Kind of."

Alex took up running and completed three marathons in eighteen months. One particular Sunday morning he took the *subway farther uptown than usual, planning to start his Central Park run on the north end rather than the south. It was during his walk from the subway station to the park entrance when the hair on the back of his neck stood up. "I stopped in the middle of the sidewalk. I didn't exactly feel scared, just totally on guard. I knew I had been here before but had no idea when. On my run, flashbacks of that night kept coming. I couldn't run fast enough."*

Story Reflections

In your journal, reflect on how you relate to Alex's story.

When your body "goes without you," how do you first recognize it's happening?

What are your physical symptoms? For example, "My body feels..."

What are your cognitive symptoms? For example, "I remember or think about _____," or "I'm foggy and completely confused."

How is your SSS overzealous, like Alex's, when you are actually safe?

Do you listen to your body or try to ignore it, pushing through to create an illusion of normalcy? In what ways has that been important in your process of surviving?

Can't Remember, Can't Forget

You can't feel safe or reclaim pleasure only through your mind. These are *sensation-al* experiences; by "sensation-al" I mean sense-based experiences that are physically sensed and emotionally perceived. In the moments your body feels unpredictable and unruly, it is not trying to betray you. *It is trying to save you.* There's a wise, self-protective part of your truest, most knowing self that senses you are pretending—professing to be okay and faking your way to fine. Much of the time your body can hold it together and keep the distressing symptoms at bay, though sometimes it can't. In her book *Heal the Body, Heal the Mind*, somatic psychologist Susanne Babbel explains, "Our bodies can become stuck in survival mode. Even when a trauma occurred so long ago that the brain has long since buried its memory, the body remembers."[31]

Like Alex, your subconscious may have more access to your trauma, specifically your need for safety, than your conscious, self-aware mind. His subconscious knew he was in the neighborhood of his perpetrator, and his body was the alarm. His SSS essentially said, "We know what happens here and we don't like it. Beware!" The mind-body disconnect happened because Alex was safe at that moment of his run, *and* it was true he was not safe three years earlier during his assault. His body was stuck in the past, which triggered a flood of thoughts and memories in the present. As Babbel writes, "Just as the body creates scar tissue to protect a wound, it also creates a web of cues to try to safeguard you from future harm."[32]

Alex's body was trying to be adaptive, meaning it was producing a behavior and sensation (hair standing up on the back of his neck) that would enable him to be in his environment with the greatest success and least risk. The neighborhood was a trigger. He didn't remember it consciously, but his body re-membered it and put the pieces of emotions and fragments of sensations, sights, and smells back together again.

Our minds work on explicit information that is stated and expressed clearly. Our bodies work on implicit information that is implied or sensed. Your survivor memories are a complex web of both. "I hadn't so much forgot as I couldn't bring myself to remember. Other things were more important," Maya Angelou sagaciously wrote in her memoir of childhood sexual abuse, *I Know Why the Caged Bird Sings*.[33]

Right now, in this moment, you are sitting in your ability to heal your sexual trauma. The importance of the body cannot be overstated when reclaiming pleasure, joy, and fulfillment. Your body is wired for touch and connection, but when those experiences are frightening rather than curative, your world becomes entirely unpredictable and unsafe. Stick with your process of cultivating awareness and understanding to prime yourself for healing what hurts.

Your work is to restore your faith in what you're made of, quite literally. What do I mean by this? We have to go back to the beginning of our perceptions, to childhood. As children, we learned about the world though our bodies. We stumbled and fell, put things in our mouths we shouldn't have, and tested the laws of nature and limits of our physicality. Then we'd fall, get up, spit out what tasted terrible, and say to ourselves more times than we can remember, "Well, I won't do that again." We are born with an inherent trust in our bodies. That's the way of the body, the language of the body. That's the way of the human spirit. That's the way of growth and transformation. And that faith in your body—listening to it and understanding what it's telling you—is a huge part of the healing process.

To help translate the language of your body, you'll learn to rely on something called the "pro-symptom approach." Yes, "pro-symptom approach" may sound clinical, but it is really just a practice in compassionate curiosity from a somatic (body-focused) perspective. Compassion is an act of sympathetic concern ("I feel *for* you") or empathetic concern ("I feel *with* you"), while curiosity engenders a strong desire to know and understand. Admittedly, this takes courage and the willingness to flip everything you're feeling on its head, to befriend in yourself that which challenges you most. But the process of asking, rather than reproaching, can change everything about how you reclaim your body and pleasure.

The pro-symptom approach begins with digging down deep to try to separate the pearl from the oyster, so to speak. It is not simply about discovering the beautiful gemstone but appreciating the manner by which it was made. The pearl can't be created without gritty sand, briny saltwater, and the slimy, messy oyster itself (which, as it turns out, is quite delicious!). As messy as you feel right now, I promise exploring your symptom (the pearl) from a perspective of compassionate curiosity will eventually produce a version of you that isn't just merely palatable, but utterly exquisite. You didn't pull your symptom out of thin air and decide to suffer. It has its purpose. Understanding your symptom will, in time, allow you to have more control of it. So, rather than your body going without you, you get to say, "Let's go together."

Your Pro-Symptom Approach to Let Your Body Speak Its Mind

Have you been asking, "What is wrong with me?" That's the wrong question. Your symptom isn't the problem. It's an external manifestation of the problem that can serve as part of the solution. But to sit with it, to feel it in your bones and be still with it? That requires your willingness to tap into its meaning, not just the pain the symptom causes. This exercise offers a chance to listen differently, from the bottom up instead of the top down. Essentially, you'll use your body (bottom) before your mind (top) to open the door to integration.

1. Sit with your feet on the ground in a place where you won't be interrupted.

2. Place your right hand on your heart and your left hand on your stomach.

3. Focus your attention on your feet and take two deep breaths.

4. Identify one sensation in your feet. Say out loud, "I feel _____ (numb, grounded, solid, tingly, etc.) in my feet."

5. Focus your attention on your legs and take two deep breaths.

6. Identify one sensation in your legs. Say out loud, "I feel _____ (strong, weak, warm, cold, etc.) in my legs."

7. Shift your focus continually upwards (from the "bottom up" through your hips, stomach, back, chest, shoulders, arms and hands, neck, face, and top of your head) and identify a sensation you are feeling in that body part.

8. After you have completed your journey from your feet to the top of your head, take three deep breaths.

9. Ask yourself, *"What is my body saying that I cannot?"*

10. Ask again. *"What is my body saying that I cannot?"*

11. Ask again. *"What is my body saying that I cannot?"*

12. Say out loud, "My body says _____. It also says _____ and _____."

13. Write your answers in your journal.

14. Do this exercise once a day.

It's important to understand how much influence your body has on your behavior, not as a flaw but as a strength. Your pro-symptom approach, which utilizes the question, "What is my body saying that I cannot?" reinforces the wisdom of your body and helps differentiate what you feel viscerally from what you believe mentally, which is most likely born of anxiety. *Polyvagal theory* (developed by Dr. Stephen Porges) offers an astute conception for healing trauma using cues from the body and nervous system—specifically the vagus nerve, which carries signals from your body to your brain and vice versa. Deemed "the science of connection," polyvagal theory[34] makes an important distinction between perception (which involves a degree of self-awareness) and neuroception (which is instinctual, reflexive, and based on triggers or cues to the nervous system). As Deb Dana, a preeminent polyvagal theory practitioner writes, "Neuroception results in gut feelings, the heart-informed feelings, the implicit feelings that move us along the continuum between safety and survival response."[35]

In other words, the process of neuroception and your SSS have made a pact to keep you safe. Trying to turn them off, ignore them, or talk yourself out of them is like trying to convince yourself to jump off a bridge without a bungee cord. You'd think, "I'm going to die if I do that!" Your body, in its survivor mode, thinks so too. "Neuroception is a wordless experience...it shapes the state, and then the state shapes the response," writes Dana.[36]

In your triggered survivor state, your response actually isn't a response at all. It's a reaction. A response demands awareness and thought; a reaction only demands emotion and exertion. You always want your SSS to show up when you need it! However, what was adaptive then, in the past, often becomes maladaptive now, in the present. The alarm goes off erroneously when, like Alex, you are actually quite safe. Your adaptive response becomes maladaptive, meaning it prevents you from making adjustments that are in your own best interest. For example, Alex couldn't have a relaxing run. These triggers from the past prompt necessary, critical reactions, but they've overstayed their welcome. In *The Body Keeps the Score*, Bessel van der Kolk notes that triggered reactions manifest in a multitude of ways and become particularly vexing. "These reactions are irrational and largely outside people's control. Intense and barely controllable urges and emotions make people feel crazy—and makes them feel they don't belong to the human race."[37]

You aren't crazy and you do belong. You're just surviving. When you lean on your body in your process of reclamation, you begin to understand that your symptoms, which so trouble you, didn't start as behavioral responses but as adaptive reactions. You didn't choose them; they chose you. And for good reason! What you perceive as evidence of your brokenness is actually proof of your power. Rather than asking yourself, "What is wrong with me?" or "Why can't I be normal?" ask your body and your symptom, "What are you trying to protect me from?" and "How do you think you are keeping me safe?"

Here is your second reminder to ask how, not why. "How" is your process of healing with self-awareness. "Why" is self-judgment, period. There may not be a logical reason in the present moment for why your body is reacting like it is. I urge you to stop chastising yourself for not being able to figure it out. Instead, *feel* it out. The goal is to teach yourself how to re-friend and befriend your body with compassionate curiosity. Part of your journey to reclaiming pleasure lives deeply in your body, and your body deserves forgiveness and inquiry, not criticism and interrogation.

Can you start to settle into the notion that your body is doing the best it can, doing what it thinks it should do, to keep you safe? Can you feel compassion for the part of yourself that hasn't listened, that goes without you, that leaves you shaky and afraid? Can you express appreciation for all the ways your body showed up for you that you mistook for betrayal? If we go back to picturing your SSS as an overbearing though well-meaning friend, and reframe neuroception as a mom with eyes in the back of her head, we get an amalgamation of a person who *just wants you to be okay*. You are that person.

Asking as a Friend: Exploring Compassionate Curiosity

In your journal, practice seeing your body as your ally, and address your body directly, as you would a trusted friend.

How did you keep me safe during my sexual trauma?

How do you think you are keeping me safe now?

What triggers frighten you most?

How do you think you react in the right (adaptive) way? Because to me, _____ doesn't feel right anymore (maladaptive).

I appreciate that you are always there for me, but if you could do _____ less, I could feel more in control.

When you react with intensity, I feel _____.

When you respond with awareness, I feel _____.

Separating the Past from the Present

Reclaiming pleasure, passion, and love starts with an appreciation for what your body has done right. You will never be asked to forgive your perpetrator, but you will be asked to forgive yourself, which starts with your body and all the ways it took care of you that you mistook for betrayal. Eros—your life force—demands your trauma find its place securely in the past so it can thrive in the present.

Separating the past from the present is the next step on your path to pleasure. When you aren't being fully alive and aware in the present, you are more firmly imprisoned in the past.[38] Being mindful, which boils down to being present without judgment, is an idea that sounds simple at face value, but as it's filtered through your experience of survivorship, mindfulness becomes more complicated. Your body will be the biggest pull to your past because *it's still trying to keep you safe.* Your job, through your awakened insight and awareness, is to push your body back into the present. When you sink into full attentiveness to then versus now, you encourage the process of separating your trauma from your body. In the same way your sexual health is you, your body is you. One cannot live or love without the other. As Babette Rothschild writes in *The Body Remembers*, "Ultimately, the main goal of trauma therapy is to relegate the trauma to its rightful place in the client's past. For that, explicit memory processes must be engaged to secure the context of the event in time and space."[39]

The time and space is then, not now. Becoming a survivor is something that *happened* to you (past tense), not something that is *happening* to you (present tense). Right now, you are safe, even if your body is telling you otherwise. Let's counter this: Just like you can feel the book or reading device in your hands as you read, you can take in your surroundings and tell your body there is nothing to be afraid of now. Try saying that out loud to your body, like you would to a friend: "There is nothing to be afraid of now." You are beginning to settle into your thriving skills to live differently and put the years of simply surviving behind you.

In addition to the intuitive prowess of your sexual health and body, engaging with your mind and having a resource of words holds a formidable position in your recovery. Don't forget: words inform our experience.[40] If you say it enough and feel it enough, in time it will be true enough. No matter how many times I share the powerful words in this mantra, I get excited for survivors—for you—to take a step closer to what you want and deserve. I heard this many years ago from one of my professors, Dr. Marti Glenn; needless to say, it stuck.

That was then, this is now.
Repeat, out loud:
That was then, this is now.
That was then, this is now.
That was then, this is now.
That was then, this is now.[41]

This is your go-to, your safety switch, your reminder of time and space, your pause button, and your handhold. The next time your body starts to go without you, pause, take a deep breath, befriend it, and ask what it needs. Then gently remind yourself, "That was then, this is now." Say it over and over until you feel your heart rate and breathing slow. It can also be used in combination with this easy grounding exercise that you can do anytime, anywhere, even in public. No one will know you're doing it.

Grounding in the Now

Now, in this moment, is your cue to go back to your body and rediscover all of the things it has done right. It is also time to appreciate its budding capacity to separate the past from the present and cultivate compassionate curiosity. You can follow these steps to ground your awareness in the present moment anytime, anyplace.

1. Sit or stand in a comfortable position, but even if you're sitting, keep your feet on the floor. (This is a somatic psychology technique to reinforce your connection to the earth and rootedness in the safe space you're claiming.)

2. Find a photo you like on your phone. It can be something that makes you feel calm, connected, or loved, or all of the above. It can be a portrait, a landscape, your dog, your friend, your daughter, a work of art by a venerated painter, or a photo of the ceramic cup you made for your dad when you were five—anything that feels, in your bones, good to look at.

3. Now, as closely as possible, inspect every element of the photo, from size to color to expression to brightness to mood. As you move across and up and down the photo, say what you are seeing. If you can say it out loud, great, but if you are in public and uncomfortable doing so, saying it to yourself works too. As an example, say, "I see a bright blue sky behind the mast of a boat. I see the brim of a man's brown hat. I see tiny yellow flowers on my mom's light green dress. I see the top of an evergreen covered in snow. I see the corner of my turned-up smile when I was four years old." When you are done listing the things you see, repeat your mantra: *That was then, this is now.*

Trauma isn't the only thing that lives in your body. Pleasure, passion, and great sex live there too. "Pleasure is the visceral, body-felt experience of well-being—it's the embodiment of happiness," says esteemed sex therapist Stella Resnick.[42]

Your body will always remember how to protect you; it needs to learn how to trust you. Chapter 4 will help you further release the past—not just the experience of your trauma, but your judgment about it as well. Eros and vivaciousness stand firmly in opposition to culpability and dispassion. Your mind and body have been waiting for this sigh of relief, this opening to the present moment and all the possibilities it holds. What comes next is a deeper exploration of how you responded to your trauma. Through this work, there will be a kind and honest reckoning of what actually happened rather than the hypercritical, self-sabotaging story you've been holding on to.

CHAPTER FOUR

Letting Yourself Off the Hook

I am done waiting. My father is long dead. He will never say the words to me. He will not make the apology. So it must be imagined. For it is in our imagination that we can dream across boundaries, deepen the narrative, and design alternative outcomes.

—Eve Ensler, *The Apology*

In all of the work you will do to move yourself through the healing process, letting yourself off the hook may be the most formidable and important. I lean on this phrase and principle so much that I've considered answering the question, "So, what do you do for a living?" with "I help people let themselves off the hook!" Yes, I am being somewhat irreverent; however, you need to hear this: *This is your survivor work.* You cannot feel empowered if you feel responsible.

The hook is deep and the process of dislodging it is messy. Unhooking yourself starts with understanding where the hook came from and how it has stayed inextricably fixed in you culturally, relationally, sexually, and physiologically. The hook originated during your trauma and has been key in placing blame where it doesn't belong. It has also disconnected you from pleasure and passion. Your perceived bad luck or poor choice of partner, party, parent, workplace, neighborhood, school, clothing, drink, drug, vacation, friend, et cetera, has magically—and erroneously—eclipsed your perpetrator's culpability.

Letting yourself off the hook works in parallel process with the big, unwieldy concept of forgiveness. Again, this is not forgiveness for your perpetrator; this is forgiveness for yourself. Letting yourself off the hook means settling into the present moment and the possibilities therein, and stopping any obsessive waves of constant self-beratement about what you should have done better, how you should have known better. There's no way to change what happened, and as the fierce feminist and legendary actor Lily Tomlin astutely proclaimed, "Forgiveness means giving up all hope for a better past."[43] Letting yourself off the hook means respecting how you made it *through* your past and being brave enough to try again, to love yourself and others in new ways without the old story sinking you.

Story: *Thanks, but No Thanks*

Gemma was one of those clients who I could immediately sense had "done her work." She talked definitively about her childhood in Ireland and how she had known, at an early age, that she preferred girls, not boys. In adulthood she settled rather easily into identifying as a lesbian. Gemma was so solid in who she was as a sexual being that I was certain our time together would not be spent discussing her sexual identity. She was a highly accomplished pianist and her presentation—stylish clothes, lustrous hair, gleaming white teeth— was picture perfect. After twenty minutes learning about her accomplished, almost heroic story of escaping poverty and religious oppression in her homeland, she switched moods sharply. "I'm screwed up and my partner is on the verge of leaving me," she said, sounding resolutely hopeless.

She explained that her five-year partnership was on its last legs after three years of no sex. She loved Dani and Dani loved her. It was a great match other than the sex. "Sex with her is just something I can't talk myself into, no matter how hard I try. My head wants to, but my body won't listen," she added.

Gemma relayed that she and Dani barely had any physical connection, even during day-to-day activities like cooking dinner, walking the dogs, or sitting on the couch. She explained, "Any kind of touch has stopped, which makes me sad because I really crave it. I'm just too scared. It's like there's an invisible force field that keeps us physically apart but still clinging to love and our life together."

"For some couples, affection stops when sex does," I responded.

We then talked through how she had been unaware that she was shutting down affection out of fear it would lead to sex. The shutdown had become so pronounced that she and Dani began sleeping in separate bedrooms. Affection came tied up in a painful, tangled ball of expectation. "I can't give her what she wants so I just shut it all down, even the hugs," Gemma explained. "I don't give myself a chance to fail. And it's clear she won't bother to ask or initiate something even as innocent as holding hands. She told me all she gets is rejection. I feel so bad for what I'm doing to her."

"It feels like you're in self-protection mode," I said. "Your intention is clearly not to hurt Dani, but for some reason sex has become scary. How about if we shelve what's happening with sex right now and talk about how it was when you first started dating?"

Gemma described sex as being good, never great. "There are some things I can't do and that was okay in the beginning. It's not anymore. She wants more than I can give her and honestly she deserves it."

"I can feel how deeply you mean that and I'm sorry you're disappointed in yourself. Actually, is 'disappointed' the right way to describe what you feel?" I asked.

"Sure, but I'd add 'furious at myself' too," Gemma said. "I've been able to figure out everything in my life, really hard things, but I can't do something so simple for Dani."

Gemma's face became almost expressionless and her body stiffened. She finally said, "I can't have sex normally. Nothing will go in."

She started crying but pushed on. "I know there is some connection, but I don't know what it is. It wasn't even that bad, I mean, my God, it was twenty years ago and whatever, I'm over it. It has to be something. That's when this all started."

Gemma told a story from her mid-teens about a sleepover at a friend's house.

"Some of our guy friends came to hang out that night and we decided to give each other massages. I was on the couch getting massaged by one guy, who I knew and trusted, and my friends were on the floor getting massaged too. I had a skirt on, and the guy started touching me through the outside of my panties. Then he pulled them over and put his finger inside me. I froze. I literally couldn't move. I didn't say anything. I didn't say 'stop.' I didn't try to joke or swat at him or say, 'Knock it off.' I did nothing."

Gemma collapsed on her own lap; the rigidity gone as she relived the confusing experience. "I'm so sorry," I said, leaning forward and touching her back. "I know how hard that was to say. You did great, honestly."

Gemma sat up quickly and yelled, "I didn't do great, I did horribly! Actually, I did worse than horribly! I said 'Thank you' because I heard my friends say it to their guys. I thanked him for it! What is wrong with me?"

I knew her traumatic past had merged with her almost perfect present not only because of the barrier her body had created, but because she asked, "What is wrong with me?" as if the experience was still happening, instead of "What was wrong with me?" when recalling an event from two decades ago. The trauma and badness of her past had seeped inescapably into the goodness of her life. Gemma cried for several more minutes and then explained that *since that time, she hadn't been able to have anything in her vagina. Not a tampon, not her fingers while masturbating, and Dani can't penetrate her with anything when they are having sex. "Dani says she needs penetration to feel close to me. It is really important to her and I literally can't do it. I hate the guy and I hate my body," she sobbed. "I just want to make Dani happy and be a normal woman."*

Story Reflections

In your journal, reflect on how you relate to Gemma's story.

Has your body shut down in a sexual way after your trauma?

Do you notice yourself feeling hopeless or hopeful for Gemma?

What other feelings best describe your response to this story?

How are you judging your response, if at all?

What parts of yourself feel solid, acceptable, or even commendable?

What parts of yourself feel shaky, unacceptable, and shameful?

Is there anything you admonish yourself for not being able to do that you think everyone else can?

Hook Out, Healing In

The depth and weight of your hook—your painful attachment to self-blame—is determined by how you judge your reaction during your sexual trauma, not typically to the sexual trauma itself. The hook is wedged in feeling complicit and responsible, even to the slightest degree. It finds its grip, in part, due to the erroneous belief that if you didn't say no, you must have meant yes.

Ironically, I discovered the significance of the hook when I realized it doesn't take over lives after stranger rape the same way it does with most survivors. (Stay with me here.) Stranger rape occurs when a survivor does not know their perpetrator. It is often depicted in the media as someone jumping out of the bushes or waiting in a car in a deserted parking lot—the typical movie and TV scenarios that give us the wrong information about how the majority of sexual trauma occurs. In chapter 1 you learned most sexual trauma is perpetrated by someone known to the survivor. Ninety-three percent of sexual abuse cases and 80 percent of sexual assaults are carried out by an acquaintance, friend, date, partner, family member, or spouse. Stranger rape happens less than 19 percent of the time.[44] In stranger rape, there is a confounding grace in survivors knowing this happened to them, rather than somehow bringing this on themselves. In these situations, the survivor perceives themselves as a bystander, not a participant.

Surviving stranger rape is equally as horrible as surviving acquaintance rape. It isn't better and it isn't worse. It's the same and it's different. However, the hook is immensely diminished or even nonexistent because the overriding responsibility is absent. Survivors of stranger rape can often more easily externalize the experience because they usually do tell someone, and likely will go a step further and report. This is in direct contrast to survivors of most sexual trauma by an acquaintance. These survivors tend to endure prolonged suffering because the experience is internalized—they typically don't tell anyone; it's become their secret.

Letting yourself off the hook requires a deep exploration of your body's response to trauma and the ways you tricked yourself into feeling culpable for what you did or did not do. As we discussed in chapter 3, your nervous system holds an important key to your recovery. Take a deep breath and try to go inside the following concept and feel it: *When you heal your trauma, you heal your nervous system. When you heal your nervous system, you heal your body, and when you heal your body, you heal your mind.*[45]

Survivors of sexual trauma have extraordinarily sensitive nervous systems, wired particularly to the nuances of relationships and the inherent expectations that live within them. Gemma was acutely attuned to Dani's intimacy cues, and rather than disappoint her with a continual string of no's, she chose to shut down connection altogether. This is a common response to unresolved sexual trauma (you'll have the opportunity to learn more about Gemma's condition and other sexual side effects of trauma in chapter 6). Why move toward something that hurts, doesn't work, or scares you? Here is a truth that probably sounds self-evident: People don't like to do things that make them anxious! So, the next time you harangue yourself for what you can't do, remember that you're most likely anxious. Your body's resistance isn't a choice; it's a systematic and systemic reaction—systematic in the way your symptoms manifest in response to the systemic (cultural) demands of moving through the world as a survivor.

Gemma's body was still reacting to *perceived* signs of danger (any type of penetration) and her mind was still holding on to the belief in her complicity (not saying "stop" and saying "thank you"). To be fully off the hook, your body and mind have to work in unison to reduce nervous system reactivity and regulate your emotional responses. Now, this word "perceived" can be tricky when trying to let yourself off the hook. "Perceived" does not mean "fake" or "not real." Through a survivor lens, "perceived" means the threat feels 100 percent true in your body and mind, but anyone with external objectivity would have a hard time identifying it. It is real to you and within you, but not factual. Once again, the perception is through the past, not the present. Acclaimed writer and spirituality educator Tara Brach calls this phenomenon "real but not true." She writes, "Yes, our beliefs and the feelings under them are real; they exist in our body and mind and have tremendous power over us. But we need to ask ourselves this: Do they match the actual, living, changing stuff of our experience in the world? In other words, are they true?"[46]

In somatic psychology, we look at perceived triggers and emotional reactions from a physiological (body-focused) vantage point. The most accurate view is through the autonomic nervous system (ANS). The ANS connects the brain, spinal cord, and organs, and is responsible for our physical and emotional states of stress and relaxation. It consists of the sympathetic nervous system (SNS) and the parasympathetic nervous system (PNS). "We can think of the autonomic nervous system as the foundation upon which our lived experience is built," suggests polyvagal theory practitioner Deb Dana: "How we move through the world—turning toward, backing away, sometimes connecting and other times isolating—is guided by the autonomic nervous system."[47]

Your SNS is responsible for alerting you to danger and preparing you for action. There is a release of adrenaline and cortisol, which is why you often feel fear and anxiety more than you think it. It is this physiological release of hormones that makes your heart race, muscles tense, and breath quicken. It is "at the ready." Your SNS is your firefighter and the survivor in you.

Your PNS is responsible for rest, relaxation, and digestion, and is modulated by the neurotransmitter acetylcholine, which downregulates and slows your heart rate and breath.[48] The PNS draws you into feelings of connection, pleasure, and safety. Your PNS is the paramedic and the thriver in you.

Picture your SNS firefighter on one side and your PNS paramedic on the other. When you are living as if the trauma of your past is still the reality of your present, you can't help but don that firefighter gear! You feel like you are constantly tamping down flames or anticipating when they might reignite. If you can't shake off the question of "Why do I still feel afraid?" know that it is your hypervigilant SNS. While trying to reason with yourself in a triggered moment is difficult, having an understanding and appreciation of how your body did what it did—and does what it does—is essential as you move away from blame and pain, and toward pleasure. Your instinct, during your trauma and now, to guard against emotional or physical pain is elicited in one of four ways that I feel Pete Walker best describes as "The Four F's."

Fight is activated when you react aggressively to a threat. You may punch, hit, kick, scratch, or yell in order to defend yourself.

Flight is activated when you react by fleeing or running away. It is also activated on a psychological level if you are constantly busying yourself to distract yourself from feeling the threat, through TV, social media, video games, etc.

Freeze is activated when you know there's no use fighting back (because you'll be overpowered) and you can't run away. You may go numb or dissociate. Many survivors describe freeze as "just waiting for it to be over."

Fawn is activated when you try to appease and subdue the situation in order to get away without being physically hurt or further injured. In essence, you talk or act your way out of additional harm.

By far, the most common reaction to sexual trauma is freeze.[49] As contrary to confrontation as freeze seems, it makes perfect sense, especially to your body. This is your body, in its full potential, taking care of you. "It is the senses being overwhelmed to the point of immobility. It is terror masked as numbness."[50] There is no time to think your way out of trauma, so your SNS sends the signal, "Don't move!" In the animal kingdom, you'd be the deer caught in headlights or the mouse playing dead.

In some instances, so much cortisol and so many pain-numbing endorphins are released that it causes dissociation. This is an extreme form of your body "going without you." Countless survivors have described dissociation as leaving their body and hovering above it, as if they were a spectator watching someone who isn't exactly themself endure the traumatic event. Here, in this moment of freeze, is when you may have forsaken your body. This is when your beautiful, powerful, caretaking body became unsafe, unacceptable, untouchable, and unlovable. And even though freeze is the most common reaction to sexual trauma, it can be exceptionally difficult to heal from, not because it occurred but because of your judgment about why it occurred. Your body didn't misread the situation—you may have misread its solution, but it wasn't your fault. Your body was doing its job protecting you from being egregiously injured. If you had fought back or run, there is no way to predict what your perpetrator may have done. Freeze is not inaction. It's fixed-state hyper-action—action with no place to go.

Freeze is also more common if you have previously experienced trauma of any kind. Specifically, freeze may be your body's default if you have found yourself in a position where you didn't have control, like during surgery, childbirth, or getting into an accident. It is also more common if you've had numerous boundary violations, even if those violations were framed as protective, like your parents never letting you close your bedroom door or having a controlling partner. What the trauma therapy community has discovered more recently is that freeze is also more common if there is a social power dynamic at play (money or power) wherein you could lose your job, career, or reputation.[51]

Like freeze, fawn is another markedly common reaction to sexual trauma. Pete Walker initiated this term in his book on recovery from childhood trauma, *Complex PTSD: From Surviving to Thriving*.[52] (If you are a childhood survivor of any type of abuse, not just sexual, this book will be a great addition to your healing repertoire.) In this sense, "fawn" means to act servilely and to placate. As an example, when Gemma said, "thank you," she fawned. In chapter 3, when Alex accepted the toast, he fawned. They went along to get along to avoid raising the suspicion of their perpetrators. If they had communicated their distress, their perpetrators may have thought they would report the incident. If this had happened, the perpetrator may have gone into self-protection mode, which ups the ante for both emotional and physical conflict.

Fawn, like freeze, is tricky to let yourself off the hook from. Not only do you have to wrestle with the idea that you didn't do anything, but you also have to come to terms with the fact that you were nice about it. You may believe you were both complicit *and* compliant, a doubly bitter pill to swallow. However, the truth is that you were smart. Not only did your body take care of you, but your mind also kicked in and demanded, "Say what you need to say to get out of here."

Sometimes the hook of the fawn response is so deep it engenders a disparaging belief about how you move through the world. It becomes a *now*, not a *then* proposition. You may have a fear that you are, at your core, manipulative. Partners, friends, family members, or coworkers may have told you that you are self-serving, that you'll say anything to get what you want. What these people don't understand is what is self-serving now was *self-saving* then. Your firefighter knew there was a blaze and was willing to do anything to put it out. There's no point in criticizing it through hindsight because you've convinced yourself it "wasn't that bad." You can't Monday morning quarterback your body's reaction to trauma. Your fawn response called on you to be nice, shrewd, and yes, perhaps manipulative in that moment. It worked well, so it makes sense that you might try it again. And again.

Now, if you truly believe being manipulative has become a problematic or endemic behavior, dislodge the hook to the extent you can and remember it was learned of necessity: *You do what you know until you know differently.* In this case, manipulation was a coping mechanism. *It saved your life.* Like the less than ideal physical reactions your body experiences, your emotions and behaviors will take time and practice to discharge and release as well. Move through what you've learned so far: bring awareness to the symptom, understand it for what it is, not what you've judged it to be, ground yourself in the present, appreciate how your body and mind came to your rescue, and begin the process of putting down all of the condemnations you've carried. The most common symptoms of freeze and fawn are:

- Being awake and conscious but unable to feel sensation

- Watching yourself as if the trauma is happening to someone else

- Having cloudy thoughts or a blank mind

- Feeling trapped

- Knowing you are afraid but not being able to make a decision about what to do

- Wanting it to stop or end, but knowing there is nothing you can do to make that happen

- Being afraid to make the situation worse

- Being nice so it ends more quickly and without additional conflict

- Saying or doing things that are socially expected like hugging or kissing goodbye, or responding to your perpetrator's text

Freeze and fawn are often mistaken as consent. They are not. They are also not a choice, but rather your nervous system's calculated response to inescapable harm. Don't forget, you are your body; your body is you. You made the best call. You did the right thing. You took care of yourself. How am I so sure? You are here and you are okay.

Four F's Reflections

Which reaction did you have during your sexual trauma(s)?

How did that reaction present itself?

How was it an effective reaction to have at that time?

Try to notice when you hear your inner judge asking, "Why didn't you...?"

Say out loud, "My reaction made the most sense."

Say out loud, "I did the best I could."

Say out loud, "My reaction saved me."

How has your perception shifted, even in the slightest degree, from blaming yourself to thanking yourself?

Unburdening yourself from feeling complicit is a momentous step away from surviving and toward thriving. Celebrate this milestone as you prepare for chapter 5, where you'll investigate concepts of shame and suffering as they pertain specifically to your survivorship. Chapter 5 also marks the end of your examination of the past. Blame and shame—and the suffering they have caused—have no place in your present, and certainly there's no room for them in your future.

CHAPTER FIVE

A New Lens on Suffering

Shame never tells the truth, it tells you you are not good enough,
the truth is you are. It tells you you have to be perfect, the truth is
you don't... For shame said you would never survive and the truth
is you are still here.

—Cleo Wade

As you continue the process of letting yourself off the hook, the world outside of misplaced blame begins to emerge. This is the final frontier for your old story. This is where the walls come down and the pieces come together—your first imagining of a beautiful mosaic, reconstructed of fragments long overdue for a second chance and new beginning. This is the last chapter in your journey to reclaiming pleasure in which you have a singular focus on looking back, your closing examination of "that was then." This does not mean, by any stretch, that you will have it all figured out, but you will have a solid foundation of awareness, insight, and tenderness to move gracefully into "this is now."

The two burdensome pillars left standing between where you are and where you want to be are suffering and shame. These are the shards and scars you've carried long enough, whether your sexual trauma happened last week or fifty years ago. Survivor suffering and shame are similar to all suffering and shame, but with their own special sauce, particularly acidic and malevolent. Your trauma didn't just happen *to* you, but *in* you. You are your body; your body is you. You are your sexuality; your sexuality is you. Suffering and shame expand in the spaces where you've disconnected from yourself. Reconnecting is about holding two truths. One: You are not perfect and you are still good. Two: You did your best, and your mind and body are wise.

Story: I'm a Traitor

Zabella and I met online. She was a yoga teacher who lived in California, but was constantly traveling to retreats or her clients' homes. The two constants in our sessions were an ever-changing backdrop of locations and her fantastic hair, a mop of tiny braids either piled on her head or splayed over her shoulders. She was a Buddhist and had studied under several acclaimed teachers in India.

During our first session, I felt a pang of insecurity, and asked myself, "What could I possibly offer this incredibly enlightened person?" And then I remembered that there's the human condition and then there's the survivor condition. There's suffering and then there's survivor suffering. Not more, not less, not harder or easier, just different.

As we began our work, it emerged that in her twelve years of soul-searching and self-actualization, talking about her sexual trauma had remained out of bounds; it was the one part of her story she couldn't share.

"What's happening now that's different?" I asked.

Zabella looked around her room distractedly but eventually settled on her screen and made eye contact. "I have another serious partner and the same thing is happening. We have good sex for several months, but once the newness wears off, sex becomes…" *Her voice trailed off. Then she concluded: "…really gross."*

She had explored numerous possibilities for what might be causing her disinterest and disgust. "I've read about women's libido and how to spice up long-term relationships, how to have better orgasms and why masturbation is important. I get all of that and I can do all of that, but that's not it. The only thing left is what happened in Spain. That was gross too, but I swear it hasn't haunted me."

Zabella recounted an experience that happened in the months following her graduation from university. She and a friend, Myra, decided to take six months to travel before returning to San Francisco to look for jobs. One of the spots they chose to stay for several weeks was Barcelona. "We picked a hotel that was pretty cheap, and it turned out to be filled with other college kids doing the same thing we were," she explained.

"We were partying with a group of people in a room down the hall from ours. I was really flirting with a guy I had noticed the day before. I remember thinking he was hot, actually too hot. He'd never choose someone like me."

She continued, explaining that she and Myra were "very wasted." They left the party and stumbled to their room. "I woke up to that guy having sex with me. I was so high. I remember he was saying disgusting things to me about what he was doing and how I liked it."

Zabella had begun crying but continued: "I just pretended to be passed out the whole time until he was done. Then I laid there and could see he was doing the same thing to Myra. She started to wake up and resisted, so he left."

She told me that she and Myra talked about what a horrible, repulsive guy he was, and told other girls in the hotel to stay away from him. She said she didn't feel like it was that big of deal because she had flirted with him. Then she asked, "What if I told him to come to our room and I just don't remember? Then it doesn't sound that bad, right?"

"Would you just walk into someone's hotel room and start having sex with them?" I asked back.

"Oh my God, no," she answered immediately.

"Exactly!" I stated. "And to answer your question, yes, it does sound that bad. It sounds like rape. It was definitely not consensual."

"You know what's crazy?" she asked, without wanting an answer. "I'm hearing you and I get it. I'll deal with that. But what is in my head is so wrong and so gross, and it's not about that, not exactly."

Her voice was angrier, and she had stopped crying. "When sex gets boring with my partner or when I masturbate, I think about or watch really bad stuff."

I took a deep breath and let that sit between us for a moment, making sure we had eye contact. "You mean forced seduction or rape fantasies?" I asked.

"Yes," she said, hugging herself as tears came again. "I'm so gross! What is wrong with me? I'm a traitor to myself and every woman who has ever been raped."

"You're not," I corrected. "You're replaying a really bad movie to try to control it, that's all. You're the director now, Zabella. Let's find a new script."

Story Reflections

In your journal, reflect on how you relate to Zabella's story.

Do you notice yourself feeling sad about the sexual trauma Zabella endured, or shocked about her rape fantasies? Or both?

In any way has your trauma informed your sexual preferences or fantasies? If so, how? How do you identify with the disgust Zabella feels about her fantasies?

How has it been important to keep your trauma and/or your sexual preferences and fantasies a secret?

What scares you most about the possibility of sharing?

What feels the most freeing?

Your Survivor Trifecta: Pain, Shame, and Suffering

Pain is an unavoidable part of being human. Feeling pain is a warning for what not to do. It's a mix of biological and emotional sensations in response to harm. Pain is your symptom, which as a survivor may look like anxiety, depression, disordered eating, chronic illness, substance abuse, or failed relationships. In contrast, suffering is an entirely psychological experience drawn from the meaning you give your pain.[53] Suffering is the secret, the brokenness, the not enough-ness. Unlike the grief from losing a loved one, remorse over getting fired, or distress about a medical diagnosis, you can't share your suffering because of what it means about you. Why would you share a piece of information that you're sure won't make people feel bad for you, but rather bad about you? You have likely convinced yourself that instead of being met with sympathy or compassion, you'll get criticism and revulsion. In this situation, you suffer in silence rather than share in fear. It doesn't make sense to risk rejection or ostracism, a confirmation of the defective person you've convinced yourself you are. It makes sense to hide your suffering, to stuff it, starve it, or numb it. People tend to attach firmly to suffering because it has nowhere to go but in.

To excavate your suffering, you have to lay it bare, unearth it, see it for what it truly is, not what you have believed it to be. From there, you have to invite others to see it too. Author and spiritual teacher Byron Katie interprets suffering as an invitation to investigate distress.[54] If you go back to your position of compassionate curiosity, you can ascertain what's perceived as factual, and then begin to examine your attachment to your story. Zabella didn't just think she had flirted, drank, and smoked her way into being raped: she convinced herself that her fantasies were a life sentence for broken relationships (you'll read more about rape and forced seduction fantasies, as well as relational symptoms, in chapter 6). Buying into her story—her perceived part in it, telling herself it wasn't a big deal—gave her body and psyche only one option, which was to repeat the pattern until it was met with reflection and benevolence. When we get a glimpse of the world beyond our story and see what our life would be like without the thought and judgment, we finally get to experience the opposite of what we have so firmly believed. "I don't let go of my thoughts. I meet them with understanding. Then they let go of me," writes Katie.[55] This is both letting yourself off the hook *and* detaching from a long-held, toxic belief system.

Think back to chapter 1 when we discussed the use of the word "victim" as opposed to "survivor." I explained my rationale for using "survivor," but also promised an exploration of the word "victim" as it pertains to a specific way of thinking, feeling, and moving through the world. As a rule, two distinct mind-sets emerge after sexual trauma: the victim and the survivor. Both a victim mind-set and a survivor mind-set have direct links to how you suffer. The victim mind-set believes no one could possibly understand the magnitude of their trauma; their pain is extraordinary, incomparable, the worst. A common victim refrain is, "I'm hurt and it's someone else's fault—then, now, and forever."

On the other hand, the survivor mind-set minimizes the trauma by believing it wasn't a big deal and telling themselves that they're fine. A common survivor refrain is, "What's my problem? I should just get over this because I played a part in it." The victim says, "This is what happened to me." The survivor says, "This is what happened." The victim sits firmly in how bad it was while the survivor sits firmly in how bad it wasn't.

These are common thoughts and feelings connected to the victim mind-set. What else comes up for you?

My sexual trauma was the worst.

Why did this happen to me?

I didn't deserve this.

What happened to me was worse than what happened to them.

No one will ever understand what I've been through.

It's too bad to talk about.

If I let go of my suffering, I won't be respected.

These are the mind-sets that come along with the survivor mode. Do you tell yourself these things?

My sexual trauma wasn't that bad.

This happened, but it is what it is.

A part of me probably deserved it.

What happened to me wasn't as bad as what happened to them.

No one cares what I've been through.

It's not bad enough to talk about.

If I let go of my suffering, I won't be accepted.

Of course, neither is entirely accurate. Like different types of sexual trauma, one mind-set is not easier to endure than the other, but both inhibit your ability to thrive. There's a healthier middle ground, a soft gray between black and white, that holds on to truth as tightly as it holds on to hope. As soon as you commit to "it was the worst" or "it wasn't that bad," you disconnect from the pride of saving yourself, as well as the belief that things will be better. And this is likely where you are right now.

The truth is, you cannot measure suffering. Trying to quantify it puts you in an untenable bind of looking out and comparing rather than looking in and caring. Believing someone else's experience was worse or better than yours doesn't change what happened to you. Aggrandizing and minimizing what *was* prevents you from feeling what *is*. It hurt—and there's hope. You suffered—and you're still worthy of love.

Reflections on Suffering

What do you feel bad about feeling bad about? What judgments are you placing on your pain?

How has the pain of your sexual trauma evolved into suffering? For example, Zabella minimized the pain of her rape, which evolved into suffering about how she can—and can't—love or have sex.

Do you identify more with the victim mind-set or survivor mind-set?

What makes holding on to one easier than the other?

How does accepting your suffering and appreciating how you survived feel as opposed to measuring it?

Beyond Suffering

If you think about your suffering as the wound, shame is the scab that never heals. You feel bad about your sexual trauma. You may even feel guilt for some small part of what transpired. But blaming yourself for your perpetrator's behavior, your body for how it reacted, or your emotions for what they've revealed is an untrue condemnation. Guilt is feeling bad because you think you *made* a mistake; shame is feeling bad because you think you *are* a mistake. Guilt is about your behavior, whereas shame is about your being.

Brené Brown's research on the general principle of shame is comprehensive and, in my estimation, unparalleled in the field of personal growth and empowerment.[56] As you move through our work on survivor shame, I believe it will be helpful to fortify it with her insights on how shame rears its head in other ways. But please do it at your own pace. There is no time line on coming home to yourself, your sexuality, and healthy relationships. Brown writes:

Shame is the intensely painful feeling or experience of believing we are flawed and therefore unworthy of love and belonging. Shame creates feelings of fear, blame, and disconnection.[57]

Survivor shame is a force of oppression—the feeling in the pit of your stomach, the racing of your heart, and the flush of your cheeks— that alerts you to danger when someone sees you or sees the you that you think you are. It sees what you aren't, what you're pretending to be, what you think everyone else is and you're not. Survivor shame makes a direct link between you and the behavior you so despise. It tries to make you believe that you are naïve, irresponsible, a drunk, a drug addict, code-pendent, a pushover, or promiscuous. *You are not your behavior.* You are a person who behaves in a way to keep surviving in the least amount of pain, as damaging as that may be. Survivor shame dissolves connection to your body and pleasure. It says, "I know what you've done," or "I know what you didn't do." It shouts, "Leave now!" In *Radical Compassion*, Tara Brach offers this wisdom: "Chronic shame severs life-giving belonging. It covers over the gold of our spirit and sends us into exile, from ourselves and from others."[58]

Your psyche guards your shame like your ribs guard your heart. It is critical to keep the things that are most precious to your survival safe. If you've learned anything in the wake of your sexual trauma, it's that keeping secrets, isolating, and disconnecting haven't helped you feel better or safer; on the contrary, it's made you feel worse and more afraid. It's not shame itself that's the problem. It's what you do to avoid shame that eventually kills a part of you.[59] As you begin to recognize your shame and understand how it is misplaced, you can start, ever so cau-tiously, to let your guard down and let yourself be seen.

Empathy and shame cannot coexist. As Brown says, "Empathy is the skill or ability to tap into our own experience in order to connect with an experience someone is relating to us."[60] Your ability to practice empathy as a survivor doesn't mean you have to share your story, but it does mean you have to share your feelings. Your feelings have been dangerous in the past, but when met with understanding (your pro-symptom approach), the "problem" begins to makes sense. From sense you make meaning and from meaning you find compassion.

Empathy is the ability to feel what someone else is feeling, not in direct correlation to their experience, but through their perspective. You don't have to experience what they've experienced to know how sadness, anger, embarrassment, or shame feels. Nor do they have to experience what you've experienced to comprehend the depth of your despair. Empathy is related through your familiarity with feelings and your courage to reveal them.

Whereas empathy is the ability to relate to what someone else is feeling, intimacy is the ability to see what someone else is showing. An easy-to-remember definition of intimacy is: "Into me, see." Intimacy is showing up in the presence of another without judging yourself, and letting others show up for you without fear of judgment. Intimacy is feeling safe and seen. And, because of your sexual trauma, it's particularly risky. Sexual assault, abuse, rape, and harassment are not one-sided stories—someone else was involved in what happened to you. Asking you to push past shame and reconnect on an intimate and sexual level is asking you to return to the scene of the crime, so to speak, to the place you were hurt most. But there's no way to move beyond shame other than to move through it, to call it out and shine a light on it at last. We know that shame begets shame.[61] It's regenerative and grows in secrecy. Intimacy is regenerative too, but it thrives in connection. Both intimacy and empathy are reciprocal processes. They aren't controlled by switches, nor do they function in a steady state. They are continual practices of courageousness and self-actualization.

Reflections on Detaching from Shame

Name it. Say, out loud, "I feel shame because _____."

What is the primary emotion you're experiencing?

Practice telling your story in the mirror. Make eye contact with yourself.

When you look into your own eyes, can you feel empathy for your experience? How do you know?

Who in your life can you share your story with? What will you say?

If the person is your sexual partner, envision being able to connect and without fear of judgment. How does that feel?

Imagine joining a survivors' support group and sharing your story. What will you say? Do you think it will be easier or harder to share with strangers? How so?

Do you think you can offer another survivor more or less compassion than you've been offering yourself? What makes you sure?

Consider sharing your survivorship in an even bigger way by supporting a social movement against sexual violence or donating your time or money to a local rape crisis center. How do you think you will feel?

Brené Brown says, "Shame corrodes the very part of us that believes we are capable of change."[62] As you move out of the past and into the present, you'll begin to remove this corrosion through an exploration of the nuanced effects of your trauma. You'll see how those live in contradiction to Eros, the essence of your life force that knows for certain change is possible.

Your reading thus far has been an investigation of the big picture, the macro experience of surviving sexual trauma. What's next is the micro version, as chapter 6 looks more closely at how trauma impacts your day-to-day emotional, physical, sexual, and relational life. Forgiving your body and emotions, letting yourself off the hook, and embracing your sexuality—inclusive of your trauma, not in spite of it or in disregard to it—is the amalgamation of your tenderness, courageousness, and capability. By looking differently at the effects of your trauma, you'll clearly see your strengths rather than your perceived weaknesses.

From your new foundation of understanding, compassion, and empathy, you can connect without the risk of losing yourself. Eros and the vitality you're beginning to touch within you translates to eroticism between you and others. As Esther Perel writes, "Eroticism challenges us to seek a different kind of resolution, to surrender to the unknown and ungraspable, and to breach the confines of the rational world."[63] Eros and your desire for more—particularly more pleasure and passion—systemically diminishes the effects of sexual trauma. What you've carried with you in your past hasn't let you dream or believe in second chances. Eros is all about second chances.

CHAPTER SIX

Uncovering Hidden Wounds

Darling, you feel heavy because you are too full of truth. Open your mouth more. Let the truth exist somewhere other than inside your body.

—Della Hicks Wilson

As you step into the exploration of your present, you're probably noticing that many of your most vexing symptoms are still palpable. Even though you have a better understanding of what happened, including how your body and mind reacted, the most entrenched parts of your trauma are not easily coaxed free. When investigating the symptoms that developed because of your sexual trauma, it is critical to return to key concepts from chapters 3 and 4: your mind and body are not trying to impair your healing, but are simply adapting to a world that feels entirely unsafe.

Throughout this chapter, you'll be presented with the most common emotional, physical, sexual, and relational consequences of sexual trauma. You'll find yourself reflected in the short stories and symptom lists, and hopefully, you'll breathe a sigh of relief that you're not alone. The effects you'll read about present differently in every person, but because of the common thread of sexual trauma, they often boil down to the same thing. Whether you're experiencing chronic pain, sexual com-pulsivity, depression, toxic relationships, or a myriad of other concerns, the distress ignites from your desire to control some *thing* that feels uncontrollable. At the core of your suffering, it's not about the thing—it's about the fear.

Emotional Impacts

Emotional dysregulation and psychological disorders are often the first to present and the last to be treated. In your survivor mind-set, you assume you should be able to handle your feelings on your own. Remember, your trauma was not a single event. If it was, the effects would have ended when the incident did. What you're feeling is less about what happened and more about how your mind got trapped in fight, flight, freeze, or fawn. Trying to manage the intensity of your emotions actually makes them more intense. As author and renowned trauma therapist Peter Levine states, "Trauma is not what happens to us, but what we hold inside in the absence of an empathetic witness."[64]

Story: *Consent at Every Step*

Hashim is Muslim and grew up in Liverpool, in the north of England. By age twenty-one, he realized he was transgender and also recognized he was queer. He used Grindr to meet men, and for several months was happier than he had ever been, exploring his sexuality and building a small group of queer friends. On one encounter, he stated his boundaries, including that anything anal had to include a condom. The partner agreed but then took off his condom without Hashim knowing, telling him afterward that he didn't like having sex that way. Hashim felt tricked and disrespected. It took him several weeks to tell a friend, with whose help he realized he'd been date raped. Shortly after, he came out to his family and shared what had happened, hoping for their support, but was subsequently rejected. He moved to Brazil to pursue his journalism career, where he lived in a van and hotels for four years, not for financial reasons but because there was nowhere that felt safe enough to stop. He experiences frequent panic attacks and has been diagnosed with generalized anxiety disorder. He feels the difference of being trans and Muslim in South America even more profoundly than in England, but his separateness has become comfortable. He hasn't tried to meet anyone since his rape. He wants to know that what he says matters in order to feel safe again.

Story Reflections

In your journal, reflect on how you relate to Hashim's story.

What feelings are most conflictual regarding your trauma? Were there aspects that you consented to and those you did not?

Do you feel afraid when you think about sex with a new partner? How so?

How does anxiety present in your day-to-day life?

How does anxiety present in your intimate relationships, or lack thereof?

Feeling Too Much or Nothing at All

In *On Being Ill*, Virginia Woolf writes, "Let a sufferer try to describe the pain in his head to a doctor and language at once runs dry."[65] I'll bet that you've tried to explain your symptoms to a doctor, a therapist, or a friend, and that it was difficult if not impossible to talk about how you felt—that your words "ran dry." This is because your sexual trauma caused a complex mixture of suffering. Each and every time you tried to explain what happened, you were forced to retouch the fear of what happened and the shame of your perceived culpability.

When you feel afraid without entirely understanding why, fear becomes an external manifestation of symptoms. From this perspective, it makes sense that trauma involving nonconsensual sex includes fear and anxiety as primary psychological indicators.[66] In fact, an overwhelming majority of survivors, 73 to 82 percent, develop anxiety symptoms, and 12 to 40 percent experience generalized anxiety.[67] Hashim experienced a manifestation of fear that lacked the "empathetic witness"[68] necessary to understand and integrate his emotions. As you begin the process of reclaiming your emotional well-being, it's important to surround yourself with people who care rather than judge. It's also essential to differentiate between fear and anxiety. This will not only deepen your self-awareness, it will encourage more agency over your thoughts and reactions.

Fear is the persistent belief in a present threat; it's in the here and now. Anxiety is the constant worry that a threat is just around the corner. Fear is, "I am scared." Anxiety is, "I'm going to be scared." Both emotions keep you stuck in a loop of disengagement with other emotions and disconnection from yourself. You may have even thought, "I literally don't know what I feel." The clinical term for this is *alexithymia*, and it is characterized by the inability to identify or describe emotions in yourself or others. The core qualities of alexithymia are diminished emotional awareness and inability to relate interpersonally and intrapersonally.[69] You most likely fluctuate between hypo-arousal, when you numb your emotions, and hyper-arousal, like Hashim, when you feel extreme emotions. Identifying feelings other than fear and anxiety is essential as you reconnect with the range of emotions you're entitled to. (For a comprehensive list of feelings, check out Dr. Marc Brackett's "Feelings Chart" in *Permission to Feel*.)[70]

Your feelings are information, not identification. You are not your symptoms, and your feelings are not permanent states. Even if the feelings you identify aren't particularly positive, they are valuable. Feeling sad, mad, or disengaged is a valid addition to your limited repertoire of being afraid. The totality of your being is not what you are feeling in a particular moment; rather, your feeling offers another opportunity to reclaim your vitality in the absence of fear.

The following list presents common emotional impacts of sexual trauma. Try not to overidentify with one symptom, but instead stay curious about its source.

Common Emotional Impacts of Sexual Trauma

Difficulty identifying emotions

Difficulty expressing emotions

Difficulty regulating emotions

Feeling out of control

Feeling disconnected

Fear of unexpectedly encountering perpetrator

Rumination

Low self-esteem

Lack of boundaries

Feeling confused

Feeling dead inside

Inability to focus

Fear of going crazy

Diminished ability to feel pleasure, joy, or relaxation[71]

Emotional Impact Reflections

Which emotional impact(s) do you identify with most?

What part of you still holds on to the impact? How do you think that's important? (For example, how does it feel safe in its habitualness even if it doesn't feel good?)

What part of you feels most ready to leave it behind?

What do you imagine freedom from emotional dysregulation will feel like?

Your emotional distress is understandable. More importantly, it is changeable. Being able to identify your feelings and create awareness around your symptoms will clear the path toward more understanding. Being gentle with yourself is key. Don't be afraid to dig deeper and explore what's under your fear—it will be undeniably complex, but ultimately you'll unearth a rich landscape of healing.

Physical Consequences

Your body has held on to so much. You may have noticed the aches, pains, deficiencies, and excesses fairly soon after your sexual trauma or not until years later. You may have made a connection between the onset of your stomach pain and harassment at work, for instance, or the urge to binge eat prior to a visit home, where abuse occurred. Perhaps the thread might feel so tenuous you've never made a connection at all. Could poor memory, substance abuse, an eating disorder, lack of coordination, or migraines be part of a bigger trauma picture? The answer is a resounding yes. It isn't always a direct shot from cause (sexual trauma) to condition (physical ailment), but it's often squarely within the line of sight. To be clear, all physical complaints need to be examined by a physician. If there is no obvious physical cause, it's important to understand that your body and the consequences it bore due to sexual trauma are grossly overlooked and undertreated. You are in *real* pain and there is a *real* reason. Many survivors are "somaticizers," meaning your body tells you something is wrong long before your mind lets you know anything is out of sorts. Your body was diminished, disrespected, and disregarded during your sexual trauma. The pain your body expresses now is its demand to have its say, including the attention and pleasure it deserves.

Story: *The Weight of Trauma*

Kasia was the result of a one-night stand, and her mother always said her dad wasn't worth knowing. She spent her childhood in a fantasy world where her dad was searching for her, ready to take her away from a life of scarcity. There was a constant rotation of men, her mom promising that the latest would be the one to rescue them. Kasia's fantasy world also involved recreating Broadway shows in her bedroom. Every Christmas she would ask to go to New York to see a performance. The Christmas she was thirteen, her mom's boyfriend at the time agreed to take her; Kasia's mom wasn't interested in going. The trip started a five-year sexually abusive relationship, one in which she felt special and wanted for the first time. It continued after the boyfriend left her mother, only ending when Kasia went to college.

In her first year on campus, Kasia gained fifty-five pounds. She had no interest in dating. She didn't want to look at herself. By the end of her junior year, she was experiencing agonizing upper back pain. Doctors said all test results were negative and that there was nothing wrong with her back, she just needed to lose weight. She remembers one saying, "Your big boobs aren't helping. Stop eating so much." None of the physicians, not even the nutritionist she sought out to help her control occasional binge eating, ever asked what prompted the weight gain. Moreover, they focused on her weight rather than her pain. Fourteen years later, when Kasia stepped into my office, she explained that she was happily married with children she adored. While she didn't entirely feel at home in her body, she accepted her size and had good sex with her husband. However, her back pain wouldn't budge. She wanted to understand and untangle the relationship between her physical pain, her occasional binge eating, and her sexual abuse.

Story Reflections

In your journal, reflect on how you relate to Kasia's story.

What physical consequences have been most difficult to manage since your trauma?

Have you ever considered that the pain in your body is connected to secrets you've held? In what ways can you start to make that connection now?

What do you dream of doing when you are free from physical pain?

Body Voices

Because of your sexual trauma, you were conditioned to feel that your body can't be trusted; you tell yourself you should have fought when you froze or run away when you fawned. It then makes sense that you would disconnect from your body as if it belongs to someone else, someone entirely untrustworthy—someone like your perpetrator. You were made to believe your body wasn't yours. But it is. And the truth lives in your body. In *The Body Never Lies*, psychologist Alice Miller writes exactingly about the disregarded language of the body after trauma, saying: "Ultimately the body will rebel. Even if it is temporarily pacified with the help of drugs, cigarettes, or medicine, it usually has the last word because it is quicker to see through self-deception than the mind. We may ignore or deride the messages of the body, but its rebellion demands to be heeded because its language is the authentic expression of our true selves and of the strength of our vitality."[72]

Your symptoms may be a constant source of pain or they may come and go. Maybe your body has found a symptom and sticks with it, or perhaps your pain meanders from here to there. Symptoms can grow more complex over time, which makes you believe they are less connected to your trauma.[73] The fewer dots you connect, the louder your symptoms scream. It takes a tremendous amount of energy to keep functioning while carrying the memory of terror.[74]

In Kasia's case and perhaps in yours, the attempt to escape pain creates more pain.[75] She ate to distract herself from her emotional pain, which created physical pain. At this point in your journey, it feels remiss not to address eating disorders specifically within the context of physical consequences of sexual trauma. In short, eating disorders and sexual trauma are highly correlated.[76] I rarely meet a survivor who does not have disordered eating or trouble controlling food and exercise. Their means of controlling their body comes down to two choices: expand or disappear. If they gain enough weight, no one will want them. If they lose enough weight, no one will see them. Both are potentially deadly attempts to create safety. This topic could warrant an entire chapter in and of itself. (For more on this, please go to "Your Allies and Resources Guide" at the end of the book, where I've listed some of my preferred eating disorder resources.)

Your ability to loosen your body's grasp on trauma is through listening to your body's truth. By returning to your pro-symptom approach, "What is my body saying that I cannot?" you enlist your emotions in support of your body. The following list of physical consequences is not exhaustive, but offers a general exploration of symptoms that will help connect the dots from your trauma to your body.

Common Physical Consequences of Sexual Trauma

Difficulty sensing physical cues like hunger, thirst, hotness, or coldness (lack of interoception)[77]

Exercise aversion

Exercise compulsivity

Anorexia

Bulimia

Binge eating

Self-harm (cutting or hitting oneself)

Poor body image

Lack of coordination/clumsiness

Poor memory (inability to recall childhood)

Stomach distress (irritable bowel syndrome, food intolerances, bloating, nausea, etc.)

Fear of needles/injections

Insomnia

Nightmares

Sleep paralysis

Tremors or uncontrollable shaking

High startle response

Physical Consequences Reflections

Which symptoms do you identify with most?

Which part of your body still feels the most connected to the past?

Which part of your body is most ready to leave the past behind?

What will freedom from the physical consequence feel like?

Healing the physical consequences of your trauma goes well beyond what you can see. A reminder, once again, that sexual trauma does not need to be violent, it only needs to be nonconsensual to cause far-reaching pain. Your ability to reclaim pleasure is less about healing the obvious wounds and more about being able to look, without shame, at the pain that's hidden. It isn't bruises, scratches, or scars that you're healing. Your work is learning to listen to your body in a new way. Only from a place of nonjudgment can you settle into relief, relaxation, and, ultimately, sexual gratification.

Sexual Repercussions

Understanding the sexual symptoms of your trauma is another element of your healing—perhaps the one most connected to pleasure—that must not just be recognized but highlighted. The reclamation of your sexuality is laced with the most personal elements of your trauma, but it is also imbued with your greatest strengths. As you recognize and acknowledge the sexual repercussions you've endured, you may actually feel a sense of relief; finally, you can release the suffering that's most hidden and often most shameful. It's time to sink more fully into trusting that the worst is over and something better is well within sight. Without the sexual scars of your past to hide, you can be wholly present for pleasure.

Story: *An Unchosen Path*

Yohan was expected to do big things with his life and never deviated from the path chosen for him. Now fifty-two years old, he's married to a woman he loves, has teenage children, has a successful career, and his life looks as perfect as planned—almost. He has a secret online life in the kink community where he shares stories of men dominating other men in bondage scenes. This secret causes him immense distress and he has tried repeatedly to stop. He identifies as straight, but can only get aroused by thinking about or watching men being dominated, even when having sex with his wife. As an adolescent, Yohan spent summers at his family's beach house, during which time he befriended a neighbor. He was twelve and the other boy was fifteen. They swam, played video games, and wrestled. After several weeks, the wrestling devolved into Yohan being bound and sodomized. He remembers being terrified but knowing he couldn't do anything to stop it. He never considered telling his parents. The abuse stopped when he was fourteen and of equal strength to the other boy. Yohan kept the secret until recently, when his wife asked him for a divorce because of their lack of sex. After four months of therapy focused on his sexual abuse, he better understands how the trauma impacted his sexual preferences, but has been unable to entirely stop his secretive online life.

Story Reflections

In your journal, reflect on how you relate to Yohan's story.

In what ways has your sexual trauma permeated your sex life?

Are there any sexual preferences or sexual obstacles that you wish you could get rid of?

Do you feel anger, shame, fear, or something else when you think about those preferences?

What will freedom from the sexual repercussion feel like?

Not Informed, Misinformed

Sexual trauma differs from other kinds of interpersonal trauma because it's not only about disregard, disrespect, manipulation, or malice—it's about sex. It's about a part of yourself that you can't separate from, and thus your understanding of who you are as a sexual being is affected. It doesn't matter whether you suffered trauma early or late in life, your sexual experiences from that moment forward were inevitably altered. Like Yohan, you may have sexual preferences that are directly related to your trauma. Perhaps you're compulsive about sex or maybe you reject it altogether. No matter how much you recognize or repress your trauma in your current sex life, your sexual trauma doesn't inform your sexuality; it misinforms it. Your sexual trauma didn't orient you; it disoriented you. To be clear, you are not gay, straight, bi, asexual, queer, kinky, or vanilla because of your trauma. There may be some aspects of what happened to you that impacts your sexuality, but that's more about unresolved trauma than sexual preference. Sexual trauma isn't sex. Sexual trauma is injustice.

Most survivors believe their relationship to sex is abnormal. I can't tell you how many times I've heard, "So, I do this weird thing where I ..." First things first, there is no "normal" in sex, only interesting. And, "weird" is a judgment. If the sex you're having is sex positive, meaning it checks the boxes for consent and pleasure, it's not only normal, it's good! Now, if the sex you're fanaticizing about or having with yourself or someone else is distressing, that's problematic. Feeling bad about sex isn't normal. It can be typical, but it's not normal.

Your sexual trauma should be the last time you ever have painful sex, emotionally or physically, but pain issues are often the sexual repercussions that feel most directly related to trauma. Vulvodynia (chronic, unexplained pain in the area around the opening of the vagina), dyspareunia (persistent and recurrent genital pain that occurs just before, during, or after intercourse), and vaginismus (pain caused by muscle spasms in the pelvic floor that make any kind of penetration painful or impossible) are common for people with vulvas and vaginas, and include pain during penetration or around the vaginal opening. Pain that occurs with erections or ejaculation is common for people with penises. As with physical symptoms, sexual pain issues should be examined by a physician. There are a variety of effective treatments, including pelvic floor therapy.

Symptoms that feel less directly related to your trauma may involve feeling bad about how much you want or don't want sex, what you fantasize about, using sex as validation, or feeling repulsed by sexual touch. In regard to the latter, if your trauma included affection or nurturance, any type of sexual experience with those qualities may feel unmanageable. Conversely, you may have become compulsive around sex, which is likely your attempt to reduce your trauma's meaning and impact. Your subconscious line of thinking goes, "If I can prove to myself that sex doesn't mean anything by having a lot of it, my sexual trauma won't mean anything either."[78]

Here's the tricky part: you may want a lot of sex to subconsciously resolve your trauma or you may want a lot of sex because that's how your body and psyche are wired. Both things can be true and absolutely neither should be pathologized. Remember, not everything about your sexuality has to do with your trauma. Forced seduction or rape fantasies are a perfect example of this. These types of fantasies are common for survivors *and* they are common for people in general. In the research for his book *Tell Me What You Want*, on the science of sexual desire, author and social psychologist Justin Lehmiller found that nearly two-thirds of the women and more than half of the men he surveyed had forced seduction fantasies. "Though women," he explained, "tend to have fantasies of this nature more often than men, they are not unique to one gender (or sexual orientation, for that matter)."[79] Several studies suggest people with sexual trauma histories have the same proportion of forced seduction fantasies as those without a trauma history, while others point to the percentage being slightly higher for those impacted by sexual trauma.[80]

Using sex to feel validated, or attaching it directly and solely to your sense of self-worth, is also relatively common.[81] Sex without self-awareness can't make you feel safe, beautiful, in control, powerful, or loved. Good sex can give you these feelings, but retraumatization can't. Remember, you are your body and your body is you; you are your sexuality and your sexuality is you. In *The Tao of the Body*, somatic psychotherapist Mary Starks Whitehouse writes, "The less the body is experienced, the more it becomes an appearance; the less reality it has, the more it must be undressed or dressed up; the less it is one's own known body, the further away it moves from anything to do with one's self."[82]

Once again, the following list is not exhaustive. You may see yourself here, or there may be more to your story. What you do or don't do, can or can't do, in regard to sex is worth understanding through two lenses: one of your sexual trauma, the other of your sexual self.

Common Sexual Repercussions of Sexual Trauma

Compulsivity with sex or pornography

Pain during sex

Vaginismus or dyspareunia (pain with vaginal penetration)

Frequent urinary tract infections

Vulvodynia (pain near or around the vaginal opening)

Low desire/libido

Feeling asexual

Easily triggered by sexual touch

Feeling numb during sex

Feeling panicked during sex

Avoiding sex

Using sex for power or control

Inability to get aroused during sex

Anorgasmia (inability to achieve orgasm)

Using sex as validation

Fear of masturbation

Fear of childbirth

Distressing sexual fantasies

Sexual Repercussions Reflections

Which symptoms do you identify with most?

How have you connected the dots from your sexual concerns to
your trauma?

What parts of your sexuality feel informed by trauma?

What parts of your sexuality feel informed by choice?

Your willingness to investigate the most sensitive impacts of your
trauma is not just praiseworthy; it's courageous. Because of your trauma,
your sexuality is complex but not weird, and certainly not irreparable.
Separating what feels innate from what feels hurtful is essential as you
make choices about who you want to be in your sexual reclamation.

Relational Effects

You want what most people want when it comes to intimate relationships. You want to feel respected, supported, and desired, and know that
your contributions to your relationships are as important as your partner's. How sexual trauma affects intimate partner relationships is
another area of study that is underserved, yet one of the most conse-
quential pain points and barriers to healing. Sexual trauma happens in

relationships—there is always another person involved—and because of this, your ability to connect is almost always impaired. The importance of cultivating relationships that hold the tension between security and passion cannot be overstated. There will be a point in the very near future where your healing is less about you, and more about you and the other person or people you have relationships with. As venerated author and couple's therapist Esther Perel states, "The quality of your life ultimately depends on the quality of your relationships."[83]

Story: *Pretty Unhappy*

Demi moved to Paris to model at age eighteen. After months of struggling, she booked a job with a high-profile photographer. This began a lengthy grooming process, during which time the photographer would buy her gifts, take her out, and book her jobs in return for sexual favors. The photographer would ask Demi to massage her, kiss her, and perform oral sex on her, after which she would give her cash or confirmation of the next job. Demi would leave and immediately vomit, shower, and try to forget. Demi is gay and the photographer was objectively attractive, yet the sex felt disgusting. During those moments, her career seemed more important than her body. Ten years later, Demi is still strikingly beautiful and gets plenty of attention from women she likes, but she cannot maintain a relationship. Sometimes she experiences flashbacks when a date merely touches her hand, while at other times she's able to maintain a relationship for several months until things get too intimate. She's afraid a partner might somehow see what she's trying to hide, so she ends it. No amount of pretty can outshine the ugliness she feels, especially when a partner expresses genuine fondness. She feels incredibly unhappy about being single. Starting therapy was her attempt to tip the scale, so togetherness finally feels better than aloneness.

Story Reflections

In your journal, reflect on how you relate to Demi's story.

What aspects of Demi's story parallel yours in regard to intimate relationships?

Does it feel unsafe to be in an intimate relationship? If yes, how so?

What factors from your trauma have impaired your ability to be in a healthy relationship? What will it be like to feel completely seen by a partner?

The Paradox of Connection

Intimacy feels both necessary and terrifying. You want it, you don't want it; you need it, you can't stand it. The push and pull makes you angrier at yourself than at the object of your affection or affliction. Perhaps when you're with your partner, all you want is to be alone. Or when you're away from your partner, all you want is to be together. Intimacy, in this vernacular, is perhaps best described as something you desire but can't tolerate. Fortunately, this paradox is solvable. That said, you can't think your way to a healthy relationship. You have to take action by showing up, knowing your truth, and perhaps even speaking it out loud.

In their seminal work for survivors of sexual abuse, *The Courage to Heal*, therapists and authors Ellen Bass and Laura Davis write, "[Survivors] may have managed short-term relationships, or even long-term ones, before they began to deal actively with the abuse. They kept their coping mechanisms intact and though depth was sacrificed, they functioned well enough."[84] Discovering what is "yours" versus what is "ours" within the context of healthy relationships is imperative as you reclaim pleasure and passion. You'll have to expose the dynamics that are at play because of "us," meaning what's happening between you and the other person involved, as opposed to the dynamics that are at play because of what's happening between you and your trauma, which is actually between you and fear.

If your relationship is founded on love, respect, and equanimity, you may be struggling because it's the *right* relationship, not the wrong one. If you still don't believe you deserve love, getting it challenges your entire sense of self. However, that conflict is within you, not the relationship. Don't reject the relationship because you believe you don't deserve it. Reject it on its own merits. Maybe the timing isn't right. Maybe you're not sexually compatible. Maybe you want different things from life. Maybe, even, your partner doesn't deserve you. It's time to drop the idiom, "It's not you, it's me," though everything can't be about your partner's faults either. Your trauma is the third party in the room. As sexy as a threesome may sound, this isn't it.

Your first experience of adoration and protection was most likely from your parents or other family members. Sexual trauma disrupts these feelings, no matter when it happens. You learned your world wasn't safe first because of your perpetrator's behavior, and second because of shame. It's difficult for you to trust others or yourself, which makes maintaining a healthy relationship a near impossibility. The ability to bond with others is called "attachment," of which there are four styles. These are secure, dismissive, anxious, and disorganized. In short, there's secure while the rest are considered insecure. In *Attached*, which explores the science of love and adult attachment, Amir Levine and Rachel Heller explain that "getting attached means that our brains become wired to seek the support of our partner by ensuring the partner's psychological and physical proximity. If our partner fails to reassure us, we are programmed to continue our attempts to achieve closeness until the partner does."[85]

It is generally true that people will keep attempting to attach (we're inherently social creatures), but some stop trying—especially those who have had their trust breached enough times. Knowing where your fear surrounding intimacy exists is your first step toward healing. Do you often feel abandoned, suffocated, dismissed, or even invisible? This is important to investigate. Your attachment style is not fixed, but again, it must be healed relationally.[86] This is another component of your reclamation that you can't merely think yourself through. Your next relationship will require independence and sovereignty of choice as an underpinning of healthy attachment. There's you *and* there's the relationship, both of which will work to restore life beyond surviving.

The following list comprises the most common relational effects of sexual trauma and serves as a gentle reminder that you didn't get hurt on your own, nor will you heal on your own. Your relationships will work in a symbiotic process to thriving, with awareness, compassion, and trust as keystones.

Common Relational Effects of Sexual Trauma

Insecure attachment style

Difficulty staying present

Erratic swings in relationship

Codependence

Fear of abandonment

Feeling misunderstood

Angry or violent outbursts

Easily triggered by words of affection

Believing sex and love cannot coexist

Confusing sex for love

Creating an unhealthy hierarchy of control (either above or beneath your partner)

Fear that affection will lead to sex

Secret keeping

Inability to communicate relational preferences

Relational Effects Reflections

Which symptoms do you identify with most?

How does it feel to know that neither you nor your partner may not be solely responsible for your relationship difficulties?

What parts of your relationships—or lack thereof—feel informed by trauma?

What parts of your relationships feel informed by fondness or love?

"Your task is not to seek love, but merely to seek and find all the barriers within yourself that you have built against it," wrote poet and theologian Rumi.[87] Your barriers make sense, but they do not make for a pleasureful or passionate life. Your walls can come down *and* you can feel safe. Safety and secure attachment aren't mutually exclusive.

Thriving insists on investigating what's being held just beneath the surface—the part you've been afraid to touch for fear of feeling too much. For a time, you concluded that the negative consequences of the known—your anxiety, pain, sexual problems, and failed relationships—were preferable to the fear of the unknown. In this case, you may have unconsciously decided it was better to have something to cling to, like your shame, a glass of wine, or a stranger's hand you didn't really want to hold, rather than the seemingly bottomless pit of the untold and uncontrollable. Your suffering held its place and served its purpose. Now it's your truth's time to shine. The following chapter sets the stage for you to put theory into practice through the unconditional pursuit of wholeness.

CHAPTER SEVEN

Engaging Control

You are afraid of surrender because you don't want to lose control. But you never had control; all you had was anxiety.

—Elizabeth Gilbert

Here you are. You've arrived at the work, your work. You have carefully excavated the past to uncover the truths and untruths of your sexual trauma. You understand where blame and shame should be placed, and how your emotions, body, relationships, and sexuality have been the bearers of your dis-ease, of not feeling safe, of not being believed or respected. You've rescripted an enormous part of what happened and can see now, in the present moment, how your symptoms have been saying all of the things you haven't been able to. From this point on, you will look forward and take steps to change what is while envisioning what can be.

The next three chapters are your practical, hands-on guide to thriving. The principles you'll be digging into were discovered through my dissertation research, *The Recovery of Sexual Health After Sexual Assault*, and have been adapted, reimagined, and restructured to address all types of sexual trauma.[88] You are about to be asked to think about, feel through, and act in response to key elements that are already present in your life, but haven't been looked at specifically through the lens of your trauma.

Your journey of reclamation begins with the exploration of the concept of *control*. You'll learn to feel more in control of your emotions, body, sexuality, and relationships, and experience increased self-efficacy in your response to fear and anxiety. Your need for control may sound glaringly obvious (of course you need to control things that have previously been out of your control!), but that's not the end of control's story or of yours. While maintaining control is a necessary first step toward safety, an erotically inspired life also demands an ample degree of vulnerability, instability, and risk. Thus, the premise of *relinquishing control* is equally as important as maintaining it. Self-protection keeps you safe, but it has a hard time letting in pleasure, let alone connection. This chapter will offer insights and practical exercises for both maintaining and relinquishing control—you'll no longer swing unmanageably between contraction and chaos. Purposefully navigating both perspectives will create a tenable and powerful equilibrium of stability and excitement, love and lust, comfort and passion.

Story: *No More Mr. Nice Guy*

Estefan never let me see him. He called me "Doc" rather than by name. This was his solution to positioning me as a nameless, faceless guide; anything else would have been too personal. We met over the phone at his request, and after our first session, I understood why. He cried several times and at least once every session throughout the duration of our work. He was sixty-two years old and had never told anyone about his sexual abuse or the sexual compulsivity that followed in adulthood. He hadn't felt anything about his trauma and had certainly never cried about it. He had no idea whether he felt sad, mad, confused, helpless, or enraged; for more than fifty years, his abuse was a nonevent. "I've been on a treadmill my whole life. I've just kept running. It was too dangerous to stop," he told me.

His early retirement pulled the plug on the treadmill, and COVID-19 further entrenched his feelings of being both alone and lonely. He was divorced with three grown children. He dated, but never felt connected or even close to in love. Estefan traveled frequently and wanted to be with a woman without too many ties to Chicago, which was where he grew up, where the abuse and compulsivity happened, and where he still lived. "I have to be able to get away whenever I want," he explained. "But I always come back and I don't know why. Honestly, there's nothing keeping me here anymore."

"Sometimes trauma pulls us back to people, places, or experiences until it feels resolved," I offered.

"How do you resolve a disgusting thing like pedophilia?" Estefan asked.

"That's not yours to resolve," I answered. "That's your perpetrator's. What you need to resolve is feeling better about the life you've lived and trust yourself to create the life you want."

Estefan grew up in an upper-middle-class family and took violin lessons at a music academy between the ages of eight and thirteen. His teacher praised him for his skills and offered special attention, often with outings for ice cream, pizza, or youth music competitions. The teacher was well liked and respected, and Estefan's parents were thrilled he had taken an interest in their son. Estefan's dad, in particular, was incredibly proud of his musical accomplishments, praising and spending more time with him, which Estefan relished. During these years, the violin teacher performed oral sex on Estefan and demanded it in return.

"It never crossed my mind to say no or scream or tell anyone. How is that possible? What was wrong with me?" he said angrily.

"Nothing," I said. "You were a child who had no idea what was happening. And, you were getting praise and attention you'd been missing. That's really confusing."

Estefan quickly switched gears and stated, "You know I'm not gay. I don't have anything against it, but I'm just not."

"I do know," I replied. "From everything I've learned about you, you're not gay. You've had sex with men as an adult as a result of your childhood abuse, not out of preference."

"That's true? You believe me?"

"That's true. And I believe you. And it's complicated. Abuse doesn't inform your sexuality; it misinforms it," I added.

Estefan cried for several minutes. We revisited the topic of his sexual experiences with men frequently over the following weeks. These "hookups," to use his words, were always transactional, not relational. "I just wanted to pay and get the release. I didn't and don't want to date a guy," he stated.

After months of working through his trauma and the reasons behind his compulsivity, we addressed the life he was longing for. Estefan was known as a nice guy, the guy you could go to for anything, the guy who would solve problems, loan money, offer his apartment, send gifts, and buy dinner. He was well aware that people took advantage of him but treasured the adoration and the "nice guy" label. His family abused his niceness, his friends always let him pay, and his dates liked his lifestyle more than they liked him.

"I just keep going back. I can't help myself," he said.

"Yes, you can," I replied. "Estefan, you're not a child anymore. You can say no. You have to say no."

The next week, Estefan told his brother he wouldn't loan him money, told his son to move out, had cut things off with the woman he was dating, and hadn't reached out to any men for hookups. Like many survivors, once he found his "no's" he was off and running with them. He was proud of himself for the first time in as long as he could remember. He felt like he was aligned with integrity rather than secrets.

"You've got your no's down pat," I said. "Now we have to work on letting your yeses back in, but in a way that feels like a choice rather than a validation of your worth."

"You know what, Doc?" he asked. "My whole life, people have told me how lucky I am. They saw my success and figured my life was great. I never felt lucky. I felt empty. I think I'm starting to feel hopeful, maybe even lucky about the next part of my life. I'm not going to let anyone take advantage of me. No more Mr. Nice Guy. That's done."

"Beautifully said," I responded. "But you can be nice. It just has to be to yourself first."

Story Reflections

In your journal, reflect on how you relate to Estefan's story.

Like Estefan, are you more able to feel for others than yourself?

Is there anything that's still scary about feeling your feelings? If so, what?

How do you feel about letting people see you sad or angry?

Do you identify with Estefan's people-pleasing qualities? Where do you notice people-pleasing most in your life?

Is your self-worth predicated on doing things for others? Did your sexual trauma inform this way of thinking? How so?

Can you imagine putting your own needs first? Name one way you can do so this week.

Control is your first step toward safety.[89] Like Estefan, you may maintain control by not allowing yourself to feel your feelings, you might people-please to avoid conflict, and perhaps you also treat your intimate interactions as transactional rather than relational. However, using control mechanisms to solely keep yourself safe limits your ability to be present in your body, sustain healthy relationships, and receive pleasure. Your control mechanisms have most likely become your coping mechanisms—if you don't feel in control, you don't feel safe. This means you're constantly self-protecting and therefore missing the best things life and love have to offer.

Control is tricky. You have to have it in order to relinquish it. You have to feel in control of your emotions to experience a full range of emotions; you have to feel in control of your relationships to have healthy relationships; you have to feel in control of sex to have great sex. When I'm working with clients, it is a hard and fast rule that I never take away their coping mechanisms until we find something better to replace them with. It's as if you've been walking with a crutch since your trauma and all of the sudden you decide, "I'm done with that." You'd fall and go back to the dysfunctional way things were, blaming yourself for not being able to will your way to change. Maintaining and relinquishing control is a daily practice, not a one-time decision.

Your work around control is not about learning to tolerate feelings of being unsafe, but rather expanding how you move through the world to experience safety differently, in the ways that exist beyond surviving. Actor and sexual assault survivor Michaela Coel, from HBO's *I May Destroy You*, explains how her need to maintain control and a sense of safety manifested: "I learned that when I am traumatized, I make a line and I say dangerous/safe. Sometimes when you stay in that mode too long, the line becomes good/bad, nice/evil, angel/devil, not me/me, friends/enemies. But the line is not real. I'm not saying remove the line, but if we understand that it isn't real, it may enable us to look at the thing that we are calling 'over there' differently. And when you acknowledge it and look at it—that enemy, that evil, that bad thing—the more you learn how to master it and temper it."[90]

Playing with the nuance of control often generates a flurry of no's, like Estefan. You may also experience periods of intense anger. Dr. Marc

Brackett, a psychologist and founder of the Yale Center for Emotional Intelligence, describes anger as a reaction to a perceived injustice.[91] Through my lens as a trauma therapist, I know that if you are feeling angry, you are healing! Being angry about an injustice means you are externalizing your anger—it is going outward toward the situation or your perpetrator—rather than inward toward yourself. Feeling angry is a step into control. Anger sits in direct opposition to minimization. It prods you to action and reclamation.

Your Reclamation Proclamation

During your trauma, you learned your needs came second and that your words—if you were able to utter them—were pointless. Part of your exploration of control includes your ability to say no and have it respected, as well as your ability to say yes and mean it. The paradox? If you don't have your no's down, your yeses are almost meaningless.[92] "No" was most likely one of your first words; no to bath time, no to coming in for dinner, no to eating your vegetables. But as you got older, especially if you were raised in a way that enforced gender roles for a girl, your no's were trained out of you as niceness and compliance became the expected norm. No matter your gender, being a "good girl" or a "good boy" isn't a viable option anymore. Most often, thriving isn't compliant and it doesn't play nice. It's dramatic, voracious, and thunderous.

As you read in Estefan's case, moving through the world always saying yes leads to codependency and feelings of powerlessness. But you'll have to watch yourself on the flip side of this equation too. An unremitting cacophony of no's can elicit feelings of isolation, immobility, anger, and self-loathing. Author and researcher Brené Brown hit the mark when she said, "Anger is a powerful catalyst but a tough lifelong companion."[93] Your thrivership is the refined and reworked middle ground of choice manifested through your body and your actions. You are in charge now. Once you settle into that truth you can settle into

Eros, which includes your desire for more pleasure, more connection, more intimacy, more joy, more love, and yes, more good sex!

Speaking Your Truth

"Speak your mind even if your voice shakes," a quote attributed to the late Supreme Court justice Ruth Bader Ginsburg, is the perfect offering for where you're going.[94] Saying no will take practice as you discover the situations in which it is your best and only answer to maintain control. Similarly, saying yes will require patience as you determine when it's necessary to relinquish control as a means of satisfying yourself, not others. You can practice this exercise on your own in a mirror, or preferably with a trusted friend or partner.

Part 1: Your only job is to say "No." Your partner's only job is to say "Yes."

1. Stand in front of your partner or a mirror (if you can't stand, sit with your feet on the floor, your back straight and chest out).

2. Look into your partner's eyes or your own eyes.

3. Take a deep breath, exhale, and say out loud, "No."

4. Your partner responds, "Yes." (If you're practicing in the mirror, imagine someone saying "Yes.")

5. Pause, take another deep breath, exhale, and repeat, "No."

6. Your partner says, "Yes."

7. Take a deep breath and respond more emphatically, "No!"

8. Your partner will respond just as emphatically, "Yes!"

9. Take another deep breath and respond, "No."

10. Your partner pleadingly responds, "Yes."

11. Continue this pattern for 30 to 60 seconds, with both you and your partner varying the inflection of your no's and yeses, from soft and

pleading to loud and demanding. If they whisper, you whisper. If they yell, you yell. Your "no" holds strong and immutable no matter their entreaty.

Intermission: Take three deep breaths in and out, then shake your arms and legs as if they had fallen asleep and you're trying to get feeling back into them. Roll your shoulders forward and back a few times to release any tension in your neck. Open and close your mouth several times and move your jaw side to side.

Part 2: Your only job is to say "Yes." Your partner's only job is to say "No."

1. Once again, look into your partner's eyes or your own eyes.

2. Take a deep breath, exhale, and say out loud, "Yes."

3. Your partner will respond, "No." (If you're practicing in the mirror, imagine someone saying "No.")

4. Continue steps 4 to 10 just like Part 1, but this time, you're the one saying "Yes" and your partner says "No."

5. Continue the pattern for 30 to 60 seconds, with both you and your partner varying the inflection of your yeses and no's, from soft and pleading to loud and demanding. Your "Yes" is for you, and a gateway to experiencing the pleasure and connection you *deserve*.

Reflections on Yeses and No's

How does saying "No" repeatedly feel?

How does saying "Yes" repeatedly feel?

Do you believe yourself when you say these words? How do you know?

When in your life, outside of your sexual trauma(s), did you not say no and wish you had?

When in your life did you say yes and were glad you did?

Identify one area of your life where you are compelled to say more no's.

Identify one area of your life where you are excited to say more yeses.

When you say no, you feel more _____.

When you say yes, you feel more _____.

There's not a single area of your life that isn't touched by control. You feel anxious and afraid when you sense a lack of control, and stuck and alone when you control too much. This paradigm will shift as you trust yourself in your sovereignty. You're stepping into Eros, your vital life force, and tuning into what feels right rather than buying into the right thing to do. You are putting your needs first. You give agency to your voice and body through your yeses and no's. The next part of your journey includes recognizing habitual patterns of control that no longer serve you, and learning to step out of them. This will feel risky, *and you will be safe.*

Taking Yourself to the Bad Movies

A hard truth of your survivorship has been the realization that fear and anxiety didn't end when your trauma did. These beliefs and behaviors live in you not only because of what happened, but also because of what you believe might happen. It isn't so much a person or situation that you're afraid of; it's uncertainty that scares you. You don't know what's going to happen. And worse, you don't trust yourself if something unexpected does. The unknown is what scares you most.

Because of your tendency to minimize and marginalize your trauma, you replay a soundtrack in your head that goes something like, "I should have known better," "How could I have been so stupid?" and "What is wrong with me?" Anxiety tells you that you're not going to be able to handle what's next, what's unknown, what's out there. Control is your handle. But it's not control of a situation you need, but rather control of yourself and belief in your inherent resiliency. When my clients are struggling with anxiety and self-doubt, I'll often ask, "Has there ever been a time in your life that you haven't taken care of yourself?" For most, the answer is no. Even if they were in an abusive relationship, they found their way out. If they were addicted to drugs, they found rehab. If they were depressed, they found therapy or were prescribed meds. And you are here reading this book—which means you are taking care of yourself! You have more control than you think.

Part of your struggle with control has been around controlling your thoughts. But the truth is, anxiety overrides cognition—you literally can't think if you're anxious. You berate yourself for your stupidity or naiveté, when it's really just anxiety. The trauma of your past lives in your body as your mind anticipates danger in the future; you're living as if the worst will happen. Living "as if" isn't thriving, it's surviving. This phenomenon of negative anticipation or "anticipatory anxiety" is called catastrophizing.[95] It's a cognitive distortion that prompts you to jump to the worst possible conclusion. When a situation is upsetting or anxiety producing but not necessarily catastrophic, you still feel like you are in the midst of crisis.[96] You anticipate in order to control, but you're controlling an aberration fueled by self-protection. You aren't safer because you anticipate, just more inhibited.

Your past gives you a skewed perception of what's happening in the present. You didn't have control, which leads you to the belief that you don't have control. Remember, *that was then, this is now*. You will feel more in control by catching the distortion through the conscious recognition that you are living "as if." One of my favorite ways to help survivors—to help you—elicit more control of anxiety is through a simple concept I learned from my therapist many years ago. I was overwhelmed and trying to explain why my fear (which was actually my catastrophizing) was rational. She said matter-of-factly, "Wow, it sounds like you're taking yourself to the bad movies."[97] It changed everything, not in that moment or even the days or weeks that followed, but after months and years of practice by literally acknowledging to myself time and time again, "I'm taking myself to the bad movies right now." I was not living in what was, but living in the anxious state of what if.

You are not a prisoner of your projections. Call them out. Name them to tame them. Once you know you're at a bad movie, switch theaters or change the channel; do whatever you need to do and use whatever personal metaphor works for you to make the conscious choice to go to a better one. Awareness precedes choice and choice precedes behavior. You must first know better to do better.[98] In time, you'll turn the projections off and feel yourself purposefully settle into the present moment, rather than into the trauma of your past or anxiety about your future. By bringing awareness to the present, you change how you think. You'll adjust your decisions to the reality of the moment and learn to trust in your abilities to keep yourself safe.

"Bad Movie" Reflections

What people, places, or situations activate your sense of being unsafe?

Are there any words or phrases that make you feel unsafe?

Are there any kinds of touch that are intolerable and scary?

Your worst-case scenario is _____.

How does your worst-case scenario align with what's actually happening?

How might sharing your "bad movie" with a trusted friend, partner, or therapist affect your ability to feel safer?

At Arm's Length

The concept of healthy boundaries is a foundation of most mental health practices. Boundaries are particularly critical for you, namely because they have been violated in the past and your desire for control is in direct response to this. In short, a boundary is anything that marks a limit to your personal dignity.[99] There's a perceptual line that gets tripped when a behavior causes emotional harm. Because your sexual trauma was both a psychological and a physical boundary violation, your mind and body must work in unison to establish your autonomy and freedom of choice.

Reclaiming pleasure—and taking steps toward a healthy sex life—requires you to amplify and enhance your voice and choice through an intricate dance of self-realization and communication. Asking for what you want and declaring what you don't want is a prerequisite to pursuing deeper intimacy and better sex. You need to feel solid not only in your words, but also in your body. Being able to control your proximity to others, as well as theirs to you, is a practice in the power of boundaries. Like your yeses and no's, and your ability to be present with "what is" rather than "what if," experimenting with proximity is another step into your empowered, erotic self.

Your Body, Your Voice

It's important to practice negotiating physical and emotional boundaries before you try to negotiate intimate or sexual ones. Feeling respected and expansive instead of dismissed and constricted allows room for playfulness, creativity, and imagination. In this exercise, you'll use your voice and body to mark limits to your integrity.

Part 1: Gestures

1. Stand across from your partner at an approximate distance of six feet.

2. Take three steps backward while your partner stands still.

3. Motion with your hand for your partner to walk forward.

4. After they take a few steps, motion for them to stop.

5. Motion for them to move backward.

6. Motion for them to stop.

7. Motion for them to move forward again. Let them walk toward you until the proximity between you and them is uncomfortable and your physical boundary feels crossed. Put your hand up for them to stop.

8. Motion for them to walk backward. When they reach your ideal proximity for comfort and safety, motion for them to stop.

Intermission: Take three deep breaths and switch roles. Your partner will now be directing you closer and farther with physical gestures.

Part 2: Voice

1. Stand across from your partner at an approximate distance of six feet.

2. Take three steps backward while your partner stands still.

3. Say to your partner, "Move back."

4. After they take a few steps, say, "Stop."

5. Say, "Come closer."

6. After they take a few steps toward you, say, "Stop."

7. Say, "Come closer" and let them proceed to a distance that feels uncomfortable and your boundary feels crossed. Say, "That's too close. Please move back."

8. As they step back and reach your ideal proximity for comfort and safety, say, "Stop."

By exploring your boundaries and having the experience of your partner respecting them, you'll more easily recognize what feels good and what doesn't and be able to use your body and voice to meet those needs. Your boundaries will become more flexible based on the situation and person you're with. You'll trust yourself to speak up and show up when you feel anxious. Instead of people-pleasing, isolating, or projecting, you'll have a well-rehearsed practice in presence and resiliency.

Your journey through control has served as an essential opening act to the element of pleasure, covered in the next chapter. Exploring pleasure is where your process of reclamation becomes more hands on, asking that you come home to your body and the expectation of more, which is the foundation of Eros. You'll discover things that are surprising but also exciting, offering a glimpse into the indispensable pieces of your most authentic sexual self.

CHAPTER EIGHT

In Pursuit of Pleasure

Any real ecstasy is a sign you are moving in the right direction—don't let any prude tell you otherwise.

—Saint Teresa of Ávila

Have you considered what you like in bed? How much space does the idea of pleasure occupy when you're considering having sex? Probably not much, which isn't close to enough! Because of your trauma, your attention has likely been focused on meeting the needs of your partner rather than yourself. To reclaim the essential facets of your sexual health, it's time to affirm pleasure as your birthright, not an afterthought. As you learn to prioritize pleasure, sex will transcend an act of physicality to become an undertaking of self-forgiveness, self-acceptance and self-empowerment. Pleasure is your outstretched hand in search of Eros, your vital life force that extends far beyond the bedroom. It's a visceral delight that sustains all of the intricacies and expanses of your life. In *Taking Sexy Back*, psychologist and professor of human sexuality Alexandra Solomon writes, "Although sex is something you (usually) experience with another person, your sexuality is yours. Your sexuality is much more than to whom you are attracted or what you do or don't do in bed."[100]

Pleasure is a principle that cannot be casually browsed or perfunctorily speed-read in your journey of reclamation. You must sink fully into its potential. Opening yourself to intimacy that feels inspired rather than shameful will solidify pleasure's deserved place in your emotional and physical evolution. Throughout this chapter you'll jump headlong and body strong into the discovery of your sexual self as the foundation from which all good sex emanates. You'll explore your most authentic turn-ons and turn-offs, how to reintegrate healthy erotic touch, and the ways in which your sexual self-efficacy translates to an overall sense of security, resiliency, and possibility.

Story: *Tacos in Bed*

Gia had lived in the Pacific Northwest for twenty years. She'd been raised by her grandmother in Mexico City with five other half-siblings, her mother unable to live with them for what she said were work reasons (her mother had a job in Texas), but Gia knew it was personal. She didn't understand it as a child, but once Gia discovered her birth was a product of rape, it made sense why her mother could barely look at her, let alone live with her. "You know, we did okay with Grandma. It was a different time. You just didn't talk about those things," she said.

Gia's mother died fifteen years ago. For the most part, Gia had made peace with how her motherless life turned out. "Deep down I believe Mom thought we were better off without her, safer with Grandma," she explained. "But when I look back, I don't believe that's true. I mean, I guess it could have been worse."

Gia was sexually active from a young age. She remembers "playing doctor" with her stepbrother, who was a year older, around age ten. She also experimented sexually with neighborhood kids, mostly girls, in her teenage years. The experimentation included kissing and fondling, but never oral or penetrative sex. She felt that what she was doing was wrong because of what her grandmother and the church said about sex—essentially that it was the "devil's work." Gia explained, "Honestly, I don't think I'm traumatized by that. I just grew up knowing sex was bad, so I assumed I must be bad for wanting it. I can't remember exactly, but I have a sense that I instigated it."

"That makes sense," I said. "I'm glad it doesn't feel traumatic and I trust you to know if it ever does. I'm sure you're aware, but lots of kids experiment sexually with kids their own age. It isn't considered abuse if your ages are within a few years of each other."

Gia nodded her head in concurrence. "Yeah, I know. It's just that sex was my way of getting attention. Everything about who I was as a sexual person was wrong, like big-time wrong," she emphasized.

Gia knew she was gay from an early age, but was also well aware that being gay wasn't an option within her community and their practice of the Christian faith. She even went so far as to marry a man at eighteen and have a baby shortly thereafter to hide the fact that she was gay. "Having sex with him was horrible, awful, and painful, even though I consented to it," she recalled.

Repeating the pattern from her childhood, she left her son with his paternal grandmother and moved to Seattle, where she could be herself. She had several relationships with women, ranging from mediocre to horrible. "I still felt I was a bad person for everything that had to do with sex, including leaving my son behind, which was the result of sex I didn't want. I let my girlfriends say and do things to me I never should have," she remarked.

"Have you ever had good sex?" I asked.

Gia sat with a blank stare for several seconds, then finally said, "No. No, I guess not." She took a deep breath and continued, "Sex was just so I didn't have to be alone. I never considered that it should be good."

"Gia, sex is about pleasure!" I stated emphatically. "It can be about being with someone, but it has to feel good first."

She and I spent the next eight weeks carefully traversing the landscape of her early traumas, as well as a significant amount of time exploring facets of her distinctive preferences for sexual and erotic pleasure. We investigated every area of her life and created her personal recipe, of sorts, that touched on sensuality, power, and comfort. It included watching burlesque performances, walking in the rain holding hands, and eating tacos in bed after having great sex. She started masturbating again, something she hadn't done in a decade, which helped translate the vitality she felt within herself to the outside world and toward the healthy intimate relationships she was craving.

"I'm telling you, Dr. Holly," she said with a smile. "In three months, I'm going to be eating tacos in bed naked. I really am. I'm serious!"

"I know, I believe you, Gia," I laughed. "I want you to appreciate how they taste, but also what they mean. You get to finally enjoy who you are as a sexual being and feel good about it."

Story Reflections

In your journal, reflect on how you relate to Gia's story.

Can you empathize with the multilayered, mutigenerational trauma Gia lived through? In what ways do you relate?

Do you notice yourself feeling particularly sad, upset, ashamed, or outraged around one aspect of her story? How does that parallel your story?

Do you have sexual preferences you've had to hide? If so, in what ways was it critical to do so?

Do you identify with feeling bad about yourself—feeling like you were a bad person—as a result of the unwanted and unsatisfactory sex you endured?

Do you feel enthusiastic or apprehensive about exploring your unique sexual preferences? In what ways? (You can feel both excited and scared at the same time—that's okay. Just write down the feelings.)

How will being resolute and empowered in your pursuit of pleasure feel? Write down one step you can take toward being sexually authentic this week.

I often encourage my clients to think of their sexual preferences as the Daintree Rainforest in Australia, the most biodiverse place on earth. A vast array of species and plants flourish in harmony, taking what they need from one another without trampling boundaries or the inherent beauty of their differences. Researcher and sex educator Emily Nagoski views sexual preferences more like a salad bar. As she says, "Take only the things that appeal to you and ignore the rest. We'll all end up with a different collection of stuff on our plates, but that's how it's supposed to work. It goes wrong only when you try to apply what you picked as right for your sexuality to someone else's sexuality."[101]

Your sexuality is an expansive terrain of pleasure, purpose, and play. Its exploration opens up your mind and body not just to better sex, but also to a better, more wholehearted life. Because of your work on control, you'll more easily settle into the safety and sanctity of your pleasure. Unlike control, the exploration of pleasure is less about feeling safe and more about feeling *good*. From this point forward, safety and consent are manifest. Now it's your time to be both curious and courageous.

Like Gia, you may not have taken time to consider what you like during consensual sex because you were too busy worrying about being left. Fear of abandonment, which is essentially a debilitating fear of being left, is significant for most survivors. Within the context of pleasure and your healing, the unvarnished truth of abandonment is this: adults can't be abandoned. They can be left, but they can't be abandoned. Babies and children or someone stuck out in the desert will die if they are physically left alone, that's true; that's a legitimate fear of abandonment. But capable, sound-minded adults, like you, won't die if a person they are in a relationship with leaves them. You might feel like you will, but you won't, I promise. The further you step into your self-worth, inclusive of pleasure, the more solid you'll feel in your autonomy. Your sexual identity is directly connected with your self-identity. Trauma hurt your sexual self-image, thus it hurt all of the ways you perceive yourself as a capable being.[102]

Sexual pleasure is your privilege. You have erroneously accepted that sex will be bad because it has been bad. That's not acceptance; it's forfeit. As author and social justice activist Sonya Renee Taylor writes, "We have accepted lackluster jobs because we were broke. We have accepted lousy partners because their presence was better than the hollow aloneness of their absence. We practice self-acceptance when we have grown tired of self-hatred but can't conceive anything beyond a paltry tolerance of ourselves. What a thin coat to wear on this weather-tossed road."[103]

No more thin coat! "Pleasure," with a big "P," comes from knowing that deep in your bones, you deserve to feel good. Little "p" "pleasure" is where you're going on your personalized journey, through your inquisitiveness and bodily sensations. You are about to discover your sexual template, which is your fundamental blueprint of how you're sexually wired. It's the flavors, colors, sounds, scenes, and adornments of your sexuality; it's the ins and outs, so to speak, of your erotic story of who, what, where, when, and how. Like the Daintree Rainforest and a salad bar, you will thrive in variety and pick what's on your plate of sexual authenticity. When you're ready to be with a partner, the goal isn't to find a perfect match to your template. That's a complete impossibility. Your sexual template is as unique as your fingerprint. It's about daring to find *compatibility*—honestly, genuinely, and unashamedly.

Discovering Your Sexual Template

Your sexual template is made up of two main components, desire and arousal. Desire is a psychological process of wanting from a place of vitality. It is a "longing for pleasure, inspired by truth," writes author and sex educator Laura Zam.[104] Desire is generated by your mind as you think about or notice what's sexy, which is almost always erotic but not necessarily sexual. Describing desire as an innate drive, as early theorists including Freud did, is problematic because it presumes self-sufficiency and independence, as if it is its own entity separate from your body and personhood.[105] Thinking that sex should just magically happen or that it's a natural thing that everyone knows how to do is erroneous, particularly if your first sexual experience was nonconsensual. Desire, like sex, is an interconnected and interdependent part of your being that fluctuates in strength relative to the context and quality of your life. When desire wanes or is nonexistent, it isn't a flaw in you. It's a flaw in the system, a system under which you experienced sexual trauma. In what world would you expect yourself to desire nonconsensual sex at worst, mediocre sex at best? It doesn't make sense. Rediscovering desire by decoding pleasure is a chance to understand not only *what* you desire, but also *how* you desire.

Arousal, on the other hand, is a physiological process of responding to a sexual or erotic cue (you may also hear it referred to as *responsive desire*). Arousal is literally what turns you on; you'll notice that you're feeling it, not thinking about it, most notably in your body. It can be subtle like butterflies in your stomach or your heart beating faster, or more overt like noticing yourself get genitally aroused through an erection or lubrication. As a survivor, arousal may be particularly confusing. It is possible to be aroused solely through touch or a sexual cue (like porn), exclusive of feeling desire. This is called *arousal nonconcordance*, and in short means that you can be turned on bodily, specifically genitally, but not experience any mental or psychological desire. You may even experience psychological aversion or disgust. A sexual cue can be sexually relevant but not appealing.[106] Arousal nonconcordance happens to most people at some point in their lives, but survivors often report this as something that happened during their trauma. You may have experienced genital lubrication or an erection even though you were terrified or repulsed. Both things can be true and neither adds any degree of fault to your story; the fault still lies entirely with your perpetrator.

It is critical to reexamine arousal from a space of control, including safety and freedom of choice, in order to embrace a full range of pleasure. Your pleasure will originate from a place of openness that is innately safe. You can't monitor or judge what feels good if you're truly going to enjoy yourself. Sex therapist and author Sheri Winston explains arousal like this: "Self-consciousness evaporates and a feeling of relaxed concentration takes over. When you're aroused, you don't need to plan or think. The arousal itself becomes your guide: you simply go where it takes you."[107]

Desire and Arousal

In this exercise, you'll investigate an expanded and scrutinized awareness of your five senses to create a mosaic of gratification intellectually, creatively, sensually, and sexually. This is the foundation of your sexual template. Be careful not to follow a culturally prescribed script about what you should like, just pay attention to what you do like. Throughout the next week as you're heading to work, walking the dog, exercising, eating, relaxing, or connecting with friends, notice what sparks desire and arousal in your mind and body. Feel free to add elements that aren't offered here (I'm your guide but you're the expert!).

Desire: "What do I find sexy?"

In your journal, answer these questions:

1. **See.** Examples: stilettos, lingerie, business suit, ripped jeans, facial hair, freckles, dancers, curvy bodies, mountains, ocean, fireplace, bubble bath, fast cars, tattoos, etc.

   When I use my sense of sight, I find _____ sexy.

2. **Smell.** Examples: vanilla, pumpkin, apples, pine, musk, leather, the woods, bubblegum, pie, cookies, smoke, perfume, cologne, soap, flowers, etc.

   When I use my sense of smell, I find _____ sexy.

3. **Touch.** Examples: silk or satin, lace, fake fur, leather, hair, skin, weights, feather, books, linen, grass, dirt, cocktail glass, paintbrush, water, etc.

   When I use my sense of touch, I find _____ sexy.

4. **Hear.** Examples: wind, deep voice, singing, music, piano, drums, waves crashing, rain, laughter, glasses clinking, confident voice, coffee brewing, engine revving, etc.

   When I use my sense of hearing, I find _____ sexy.

5. **Taste.** Examples: red meat, cake, avocado, martini, wine, prosecco, mint, berries, ice cream, olives, oysters, olives, chocolate, pancakes, tacos, tapas, etc.

   When I use my sense of taste, I find _____ sexy.

Now, in your journal, write your observations about what you find sexy.

Arousal: "What turns me on?"

In your journal, answer these questions:

1. **See.** Examples: myself in lingerie, a stranger in a tight T-shirt, people kissing on the beach, people having sex (movies, pornography), chivalry, confidence, a woman in heels, a man's rough hands, etc.

   When I use my sense of sight, I find _____ arousing.

2. **Smell.** Examples: my perfume, a stranger's cologne/perfume, my partner after a shower, candles burning, crisp air, incense, roses, body odor, muskiness, etc.

   When I use my sense of smell, I find _____ arousing.

3. **Touch.** Examples: sand in my toes, my hair, my partner's breasts, satin on my skin, lying outside naked, spanking, unzipping tight jeans, not wearing underwear, etc.

   When I use my sense of touch, I find _____ arousing.

4. **Hear.** Examples: a stranger complimenting me, a stranger catcalling me, my partner objectifying me, loud music, soft music, kissing sounds, sex sounds, dirty talk, the buzz of a sex toy, etc.

   When I use my sense of hearing, I find _____ arousing.

5. **Taste.** Examples: drinking a martini, feeding my partner chocolate, my partner's lips, eating pizza naked in bed, licking an ice cream cone, sipping champagne, etc.

   When I use my sense of taste, I find _____ arousing.

Now, in your journal, write about your observations of what turns you on.

Reflections on Your Sexual Template

1. How did it feel to approach your sexuality somatically—from your senses and with curiosity?

2. Did you notice judgment—worrying about what others would think or if you were normal—running through your mind? How so?

3. Did you notice any themes to your answers, such as sensuality, romance, power, comfort, overt sexuality, outdoorsy, elegant, light, dark, cozy, open?

4. What are three things you learned about your desire—not the answers specifically, but what meaning the answers provide? In other words, how do your answers within the five desire categories connect?

5. What are three things you learned about what arouses you—not the answers themselves, but what meaning the answers provide? How do your answers within the five arousal categories connect?

It is likely you have never taken the time to fully investigate the core essences of your sexuality. This isn't easy—and you did it (see, you *can* do hard things)! It demands a stance of self-worth and affirmation of pleasure, all through a lens of sex positivity. From here, you'll step out of your head and into your body for a hands-on exploration of pleasure, because good sex starts with self-love.

The Pleasure Is Yours

Through decoding your sexual template, you have a solid understanding of what excites you. You know whether, for example, romance and sensuality are important to you, or whether power and more overt sexiness light your fire. You may have also stumbled on some things that definitely don't excite you, but quite the opposite. For example, you may have had the realization that dirty talk, cologne, or facial hair is a *trigger*, or something that has a direct correlation to your sexual trauma. Decoding your sexual template is mostly about understanding and accepting what you want, but it is also about being keenly aware of what to avoid. Embrace these unique aspects of your sexuality as tightly as you embrace all others. They are not bad; they are just true. No more denying, no more minimizing, no more pushing through—the pleasure, with boundaries, is yours to have.

Before you get started, it's important to understand that while the core aspects of your sexual template will most likely stay constant, the details may change. Actually, they probably will change depending on things like what stage of life you're in, how healthy your relationships are, how your overall health is, what your stress level is like, and even where you are in your monthly cycle if you menstruate. Don't let this throw you. Changes in what and how you want are normal and natural. Your pleasure now exists in a safe space that you can pursue rather than retreat from. You can use your yeses and no's to accept or dismiss what's offered. Also, you should know that your desire and arousal may not follow a linear path, meaning desire does not necessarily have to precede arousal. Because the mere act of wanting (desire) felt tenuous or even scary after your trauma, you may have trouble conjuring up things that excite you. Rather than feeling stuck or frustrated with yourself for not wanting sex, go for arousal first; go to your body, go to what feels good. Desire often appears when you finally have sex worth wanting.[108] Sex worth wanting has to be generated by a self that feels deserving. Thus, the intention to have good sex must start with you.

Awareness and curiosity are two of the most vital principles you can embrace while reclaiming your sexual pleasure. Be patient with yourself. The effects of your trauma didn't manifest in a day, nor will they vanish in a day. They may not (and will probably not) ever completely disappear. They'll most likely exist as a shadow that you are aware of and now have tools to manage. You get to decide what to step away from or shine light on. Pleasure is your flashlight, your beacon, and your sunshine. When you learn to feel good about sex, it's harder to feel bad while having it. Similar to decoding your sexual template, your reclamation of pleasure starts with your body. But rather than focusing on your senses, you'll focus on sensation.

"Having sex with yourself is your most powerful recovery tool," writes author and activist Staci Haines on healing from sexual abuse.[109] Call it masturbation, self-pleasure, touching yourself, or having solo sex; whatever you decide, it is paramount to your healing and ability to sustain long-term, satisfying relationships. Only through self-pleasure can you practice being present rather than anxious or numb. Being alone awards an opportunity to step out of your critical observer, judgmental mind—your perfectionist, performer, and people-pleaser—to be present with yourself in order to experience all of the feel-good feels. You'll further practice moving away from performance and into pleasure in chapter 9 through partnered exercises. Sex, from here forward, is not defined by your genitals, but by your whole body. You'll think about the entirety of your physicality, head to toe, as possibilities for pleasure.

In the exercise that follows, you won't be going directly toward orgasm, at least not at first and certainly not as a sole destination. Of course, orgasms are great. They are good for your health—improved sleep, better immune function, stronger pelvic floor, better mood, and reduced stress, among other benefits—and you deserve to have them if they are available to you, but you don't have to have them to have good sex. Orgasms are an option, not a requirement. As you reintroduce pleasure to your path toward healthy sexuality, it's imperative that you don't feel frustrated by something you aren't achieving. It's equally important that you don't step back into your survivor story about being broken and unfixable. You are well on your way to feeling authentically whole. There is nothing to achieve here. All you need to do is feel the sensations that arise.

Pioneering Self-Pleasure

Take thirty minutes two times per week to initiate a self-pleasure session. Once you feel comfortable touching your entire body and know what feels good, you can proceed toward the possibility of orgasm if you'd like. Pay attention to where you are, what position you're in, and what you're fantasizing about, namely what you're imagining, watching, reading, or listening to. Feel free to use fantasy or you can simply stay focused on bodily sensations. Anything you find arousing is fine as long as is it's not retraumatizing, meaning it's not giving you feelings of shame or anxiety. Remember your discoveries from decoding your sexual template and stay away from potential triggers. Additionally, make sure to switch up the place (bed, couch, bathroom, etc.), position (lying on your back, stomach, or side, or sitting or standing), and content of your fantasies (rough sex, sensual sex, gay sex, multiple partner sex, sex with strangers, etc.). Masturbating different ways will encourage your erotic flexibility in order to ensure there's an array of pleasure on the menu rather than just one or two items.

1. Create an environment that is safe, private, and comfortable.

2. Add erotic elements to your environment that are part of your sexual template, like candles, baths, flowers, handcuffs, or incense.

3. Purposefully decide what to wear, like lingerie, a T-shirt, a cozy sweater, or nothing at all. If you decide to wear something, make sure you have easy access to all parts of your body.

4. Begin exploring your body and preferences for touch, including all parts of your body from the top of your head to your toes.

5. Try various options for types of touch. Do you like lighter touch, tickles or taps, or a firmer grip that feels more like a massage?

6. Go slowly. Go slowly. Go slowly.

7. Linger on your genitals. If you have a penis and scrotum, experiment with various grips, rhythm, and pressure. If you have a vulva and vagina, notice whether one side of your labia is more sensitive than the other, as well as your preference for clitoral stimulation (the

upper left quadrant of the clitoris is generally the most sensitive). Consider whether penetration with your finger would feel good, or whether penetration isn't necessary for your full experience of pleasure. (After week one, if orgasm is an option, feel free to go there.)

8. Move your hands away from your genitals and place them back on another erogenous zone, whether it's your breasts, hips, scalp, feet, butt, or earlobes, for example.

9. Bring your hands back to an area of your body where touch felt pleasurable but not sexual, and touch yourself for a minute or two.

10. Wrap your arms around yourself for a hug of appreciation and acceptance. Take your time getting up and reintegrating back into your day (or this can be an ideal way to fall asleep, if that feels appropriate).

Self-Pleasure Reflections

1. Were you able to approach this exercise from a place of curiosity and nonjudgment? How do you know?

2. If you noticed stumbling blocks, what were they? For example, privacy or body-image concerns, or fear of not doing it right?

3. What was the most exciting part of this exercise?

4. What part of this exercise made you anxious, if any?

5. Did you feel like you could maintain and relinquish control of your self-pleasure? In certain moments could you be more self-directed, and in others could you let your hands and body go where they chose?

6. How has self-pleasure changed for the better since experiencing your trauma?

7. What are you excited about having discovered within your self-pleasure practice, and is there anything you are still excited to discover?

Reclaiming pleasure, which starts with reclaiming your body, moves sex out of the category of something you are doing to who you are becoming. "Being yourself makes your entire life better, sexier, and more livable—that's a fact," writes sex educator Gigi Engle in her memoir, *All the F*cking Mistakes.*[110]

Your definition of sex has necessarily shifted from anxiety provoking to entirely within your control, inclusive of pleasure. You are an expert on you—your likes, dislikes, needs, and desires. Chapter 9 asks you to stretch further out of your head and into your body through both awareness and exercises that add connection to your formula of reclamation. Connection, like control and pleasure, has both emotional and physical attributes, and is essential to having good sex and healthy relationships. Cultivating connection is key as you learn to trust and engender a true sense of belonging.

CHAPTER NINE

Creating Connection

Sex is about connection. It's about the ways we connect with the life force, with others, and with ourselves. Each of us is connected to everyone and everything around us.

—Sheri Winston

Daring to create connection is the last hurdle in coming home to your-self—this is your work on partnership, collaboration, and interdependency. There have been aspects of your life that were too dangerous to connect with, including self-trust ("I made a bad decision"), your body ("It betrayed me"), and intimacy ("Others have the power to hurt me"). Now, as you feel yourself another step closer to thriving, you'll notice a strong desire for togetherness because your sense of otherness is crumbling. Being a survivor has made you different than other people in some ways, but it certainly hasn't made you unlovable. Quite the contrary. Being a survivor has made you more lovable—the suffering you've endured gives you a different type of vision and more acute senses, both of which radiate compassion and empathy. People are drawn to you because they feel understood and safe. Now it's time to extend that sense of safety and feelings of compassion to yourself, through connection. As trauma researcher Stephen Porges states, "Healing doesn't come from a lack of threat; it comes from connection."[111]

Healthy relationships can only take shape when reciprocity exists, when what we need and ask for is offered, and when the qualities that are finally shining through us are reflected back. Connection is about giving and getting. It's about being spacious, communicative, and empathetic. It's about you and other, other and you. Connection, at its core, takes risk. To be connected you must be vulnerable; vulnerability is the high art of connection. Throughout this chapter, you'll practice controlled, pleasure-focused vulnerability with others. You can choose to enact the exercises in a way that's platonic, romantic, or sexual, or preferably a little of each. As with each aspect of the intimacy you're reclaiming, the choice is yours regarding where, when, how, and who to include. You'll use your mind and body to reengage with your intuition, imagination, and wisdom to transform connection from something that was once risky to a condition that's absolutely requisite.

Story: *Finding Home*

Ryleigh's life seemed enviable. She worked as a gear tester for a leading outdoor sports equipment company, traveling internationally to the world's most remote and beautiful destinations. She ice-climbed, dog-sledded, mountain-biked, and whitewater-rafted. She had a tiny apartment in Sydney, Australia, but was only there for corporate meetings. "I literally can't be still," she explained within the first five minutes of our session.

I heard both excitement and sadness in her voice, and replied, "That sounds complicated."

She quickly retorted, "It's way simpler than staying put and being in a relationship. It's just me and nature. I don't have to answer to anyone."

"That's true," I said. "But you also don't have anyone to listen to or listen to you."

Ryleigh came to therapy because she had experienced increased anxiety in the past six months, including several panic attacks. She wondered whether her constant travel was part of the problem, and if in some way it was tied to sexual trauma from her past. She was taking greater risks both in the activities themselves and by hitchhiking, going out alone at night, and requesting to work in places that were dangerous.

"How has it been important to spend so much time alone and isolated?" I asked.

"I'm definitely trying to prove something to myself, but I don't know what," she answered. "But lately I've been feeling more scared than capable. I know I'm making bad decisions."

Ryleigh and I dug back through her past to figure out when being outdoors went from a passion to an obsession. We also explored her familial, platonic, and romantic relationships, and tried to determine at what point those took less priority than being alone. "I knew my sexual trauma has been lingering in me, somewhere, but not until now did I realize what a huge effect it had on my life. I stopped staying still after I was raped," she concluded.

When she was twenty, Ryleigh had been on a day hike in southern Australia. She met a guy on the trail, and they began talking and decided to hike together. At the end of the hike, they went into a public restroom to clean up. She said she was excited about the possibility of a kiss before they headed to their cars to drive home. Her excitement quickly turned to terror as he pushed her into a bathroom stall and raped her.

"It was like he was two different guys," she recalled. "The nice guy on the hike and a monster in the restroom."

"I am so sorry that happened to you. I'm glad you're mostly okay," I said. "It's interesting; some survivors get as far away from things associated with their trauma as possible. But others, like you, run right toward them. Your constant wilderness journeys are a reenactment of sorts. You symbolically return to the scene of the crime in hopes of a different outcome."

Ryleigh answered, "The last six months have let me know, loud and clear, that there isn't one. I can't shake this feeling. I'm scared and lonely, not just alone."

Our next few months were spent connecting her trauma to her relationship fears, what it meant to stay still, to be connected, reliant on, and reliable to a partner. She completed her sexual template and then started imagining what her ideal relationship might look like. She wrote pages upon pages in her journal. She also told her company she wanted to travel less. The risk she had been creating as a solution was only another problem, and one that she needed to solve differently.

Our work had concluded about two months before I received an email that read, in part, "I cannot believe I'm writing to say I am happy at home. I moved out of my city apartment to a country cottage and even have a garden. Nature is in my backyard and somehow it works. I have not traveled in six months. My parents visited, which hasn't happened in years. I'd always go to them and leave within a day or two. I joined a rowing club and have made a few friends. Well, to be totally honest, I've made two friends who are men, and both are interested in me and I'm interested in them. It's nothing yet, just talking and being outside together, but I am open to what comes next. I'm imagining a normal date, in a restaurant, and at some point, if it feels right, inviting them home. I finally have a home and life I'm attached to. I'm taking baby steps toward a potential partner that feels safe and solid too."

I wrote back and said, "Ah, there it is, there you are! Welcome home to yourself. Ryleigh, I'm so proud of you. You know you don't have to completely stop moving, you just have to move toward connection. Thank you for staying connected with me. I look forward to hearing about who the next lucky person is."

Story Reflections

In your journal, reflect on how you relate to Ryleigh's story.

Does your sexual trauma make it difficult to connect with people?
In what way?

Is there any element of reenactment—something you're trying to
solve from your trauma—that lingers in your present relationships
(or lack of relationships)?

What do you believe is your biggest hurdle to finding a meaningful
intimate relationship?

What are three qualities you need in your next intimate relationship?

This week, take time to generate one of those qualities in yourself.
For example, if trust is one quality you need, make a small promise
to yourself every day and keep it (do a three-minute morning
meditation, spend fifteen minutes outside, connect with a friend,
drink eight glasses of water, etc.).

The principles of connection show us that most people are only as
needy as their unmet needs.[112] Bonding becomes an act of hopeful
expectation as you rely on others to meet your proximal, emotional, and
sexual requirements. If your needs aren't met occasionally, as happens in
all relationships, you'll ask again with the hopeful expectation of a better
outcome. If your needs aren't met time after time, you'll stop asking.
Daring to connect, like Ryleigh, happens through a series of belief shifts
and subsequent behavior changes. She put her faith in vulnerability,
which meant staying put and sitting with her pain rather than constantly
running from it. She became an expert at opening up *and* creating
healthy boundaries. Ryleigh no longer tries to avoid her feelings, and she
knows that when she feels them, she can handle them. Connection, at
its best, gives and takes in equal measure. If you're completely self-
protected, you can't be connected. To connect, you have to dare to try

again. In *The Gifts of Imperfection*, Brené Brown defines connection as the energy that exists between people when they feel seen, heard, and valued, and when they derive sustenance and strength from relationships.[113] Connection and your sense of worthiness can and must coexist.

Of your three principles of thriving after sexual trauma—control, pleasure, and connection—connection is undoubtedly the most well researched and empirically supported. Many studies suggest that connection with others, including friends, family, intimate partners, and community, is imperative to your recovery, including regaining sexual health. Not only does connection play a central role in breaking patterns in the symptoms you experience, but also the physical and psychological stress you've endured will diminish as you develop coping mechanisms that involve others.[114] Connection's primacy in your ability to reclaim all that you've lost and deserve is absolute.

The intimate relationship you're looking for won't flourish by being overconnected or unhealthily codependent. It's not, "If you're sad, I'm sad. If you're mad, I'm mad. I live only as a reflection of you." Nor will it blossom through under connection or your complete autonomy. It can't be, "We can be together but stay in your lane. Don't need too much and don't ask me to be vulnerable." It's the inimitable middle ground you're aiming for, which feels like, "I need you and you need me, *and* I'm solid in myself." All the energy you put into self-protection will be entirely at odds with thriving. You won't have to try so hard anymore. It's not about healing an old wound or fixing something, but rather daring to experience something profound in the presence of another.

Embracing Eros

Eros, the vitality and desire that lives in you, grows in multiplicity. It is self-generated but not selfish. It intensifies in connection to others, to purpose, and to pleasure. When you feel connected, you want more connection. This notion applies to good sex as well; the more you have, the more you want. Sex begets sex! The reasons for this are both physiological and psychological. On the physiological front, you get a euphoric hit of dopamine, endorphins, and oxytocin, the "cuddle hormone." On the emotional front, you experience consideration, adoration, mutuality, and respect. Connecting through good sex requires intentionality and presence. Remember what you learned about your autonomic nervous system (ANS), the firefighter and paramedic? You can't be anxious and relaxed at the same time.[115] It's a physiological impossibility, and, entirely relevant to your work at this stage of your journey, an erotic impossibility. You can—and will—be excited about good sex, but you can't be anxious about it. Being intentional in your desire for pleasure and connection is where you're headed.

Your sexual and erotic health exists in a space far beyond sex's functionality. The act itself is well within your control and the pleasure you crave is at your fingertips. The expansiveness of sex, the quality that shifts it from a thing you do to the person you are, is only accessed through connection. Connecting through good sex requires a mind-body dance of reciprocity and attunement. You and your partner have to be aligned, attuned, and in harmony about your purpose. Attunement puts forth the intention of recognizing, understanding, and engaging with another person's emotional state. Venerated couples' therapists John and Julie Gottman define attunement as "a special kind of listening."[116] For you, as a thriver, it's especially important that attunement happens in a safe space with a trusted partner to build and protect the connection you're creating.

A lack of attunement, and thus a lack of connection, often boils down to a singular focus on performance. Worrying about performance is where connection unravels. Settling into pleasure is where connection tethers. Fear of judgment about your body, what it looks like, smells like, tastes like, and sounds like, as well as concerns about your sexual abilities, including how long you'll last, what feats you can pull off or positions you can achieve, can prod you out of the present and pleasurable moment! Performance lives out there, beyond what is happening in the here and now. Your inclination to perform during sex is partially a result of your survivorship, namely not feeling worthy of pleasure and too unsafe to deeply connect, as well as a by-product of the society in which you've been raised. In most Western cultures, sex is portrayed as happening between people with impossibly "perfect" bodies who can last for hours and perform tricks of jaw-dropping finesse while moaning loudly, using dirty talk, squirting, or faking orgasms, among dozens of other acts, rather than the realities of sex. They follow a script of what's supposed to be sexy. What happens in rom-coms, steamy movies, romance novels, and pornography are performances. None of these forms of entertainment are particularly bad, but they're also not particularly real. To feel the healing power of your sexuality, you have to be yourself, not a performer. The intentional, authentic you is the sexiest you.

Your Pleasure Connection

As you reimagine what healthy connection looks and feels like, you'll recommit to pleasure by letting go of performance. This first exercise is meant to be playful and lighthearted, so have fun with it. You can do it clothed or naked.

1. Ask your partner to share one way they know they perform sexually.

2. Share one way you know you perform sexually.

3. Agree to mutually initiate an act of sexual performance for one minute. Play up and exaggerate sounds, positions, and moves.

4. Laugh! That should have been funny and a bit rowdy.

5. Embrace and take three deep breaths.

6. Ask your partner to share one way they experience pleasure sexually.

7. Share one way you experience pleasure sexually.

8. Agree to mutually initiate an act of sexual pleasure for one minute.

9. Embrace and take three deep breaths.

Reflections on Pleasure vs. Performance

For this second exercise, use your journal to record your thoughts and observations.

How are you aware that you perform during sex?

What do you get out of performing?

What do you lose?

When you notice yourself performing, whose erotic story are you subscribing to? Is it yours, your partner's, or society's?

How are you aware that you experience pleasure during sex?

How do you offer pleasure?

How do you receive pleasure?

In what ways does focusing on pleasure enable you to feel more connected?

By stepping into pleasure and out of performance, you create an opportunity to connect in the present moment, not in the sorrow of your past sexual experiences or with apprehension about those in your future. The dissolution of performance gets you out of your head and into your body, the exquisite space where connection proliferates. Author and sex educator Sheri Winston describes the power of erotic connection like this: "When you deeply and truly own your own sexuality, you gain the power to break free from the blockages of old programming, celebrate your own and your partners' pleasure, and become a virtuoso of erotic expression."[117]

Sex, Woven with Intention

You know that all sex is good sex as long as it's consensual and pleasurable, but what does it take to make good sex great? What lives beyond consent and pleasure? For most people, the answer is connection—to their body, their desires, and a partner. Here's a sex therapy secret that is completely contrary to what the performance-based, romance-laden scripts have shown you: great sex is often planned sex. It's sex that utilizes preparation to increase passion. Connected sex, meaning sex that leans on attunement, validation, and reciprocity, doesn't often happen in swept-off-your-feet, spontaneous sparks, but rather in moments of anticipation and communication. Planning what you want to do and talking with your partner about it is an essential part of your reclamation of great sex. Though you have honed your ability to maintain and relinquish control, it's probably true that at least in the present time, you'll feel more open to pleasure and connection if you know where sex is going. You may feel differently in the future, but for right now, let preparation, communication, anticipation, and imagination be your keys to passion.

There is a practice in sexuality that beautifully synthesizes control, pleasure, and connection. It centers on the cultivation of the present moment rather than the past or future ("That was then, this is now"; no "bad movie" projections), while letting go of judgment (you've let yourself off the hook), and prioritizing authenticity and vulnerability. It's the sexual iteration of a mindfulness-based practice, one that places emphasis on attunement instead of orgasms. We're talking about tantra. *Tantra* is a Sanskrit word that translates to "loom" or "weave." It can be a spiritual practice, but it doesn't have to be. It can also include extended lovemaking sessions and acrobatic positions, but it doesn't have to. Tantra's key principle is *union*, a weave of self with self or self with other. Tantra is your passageway to passion, not necessarily through lust but rather through intimacy. When you practice tantric sex, there's no past to draw conclusions from, no future to plan for. It's a constant discovery where you're always in wonder. Tantra is a perpetual love affair and never-ending honeymoon.[118] "In tantra, planning and preparation are foreplay," writes sex educator Barbara Carrellas in *Urban Tantra: Sacred Sex for the Twenty-First Century*. "Rather than making sex seem contrived, artificial, and unsexy, preparation and planning help build erotic energy to share with a partner."[119]

I use tantra with clients, including both individuals and couples, when everything else they've tried to do to fix their sex lives has failed. Tantra strips sex bare and allows you to start again, from a place of openness and curiosity. There's literally no room for performance or self-criticism if you follow the plan. Yes, it is slow, but it's never boring. On the contrary, its deliberateness actually generates desire. Hear this: you don't have to be in the mood for sex for sex to be great. Tantra is the mood. All you need is a willingness to connect and the resolve to completely deconstruct what sex has been in order to make it better.

As eager as you are to get started, it's important to consider your relationship to giving and receiving before settling in. Great sex is a pairing of what you give and what you get, always within the realm of your own permission giving and limitation setting. Your sexual trauma was entirely about having something taken from you. Tantra gives you the chance to flip the script through an abundance of offering and receptivity. Similar to your inability to be anxious and relaxed at the same time, it's also impossible to fully give and receive at the same time. Your brain and body are not multitaskers when it comes to sex. Your reclamation of safe, pleasurable, and connected sex demands your full attention. As an example, the "69" position is often fun and fantastic in its own right, but it's hard to entirely receive pleasure when you're focused on giving it and vice versa. Thus, during your first experience with tantra, you'll notice a division of giving and receiving, which is quite intentional. If you're in the receiving position, it allows you to relax and accept. If you're in the giving position, it allows you to attune and arouse. *And*, many people get very turned on by their partner's arousal; for some, it's actually the thing that excites them most. The following tantric exercise is in no way one-sided, but it is of one intent: connection.

The Weave

This exercise is based on Masters and Johnson's sensate focus protocol, which works by refocusing participants on their own sensory perceptions and sensuality, instead of goal-oriented sexual behavior. I've adapted it through sexual trauma and somatic psychology lenses.[120] Set aside twenty to thirty minutes one to two times per week for eight weeks. Each week you'll add another layer of eroticism to the protocol, from a foundation of massage, moving toward more sexual and genital-based touch, as well as penetration if it is desired (vaginal, anal, or both). For week one, no genital touch is allowed—no breasts, butt, vulva, penis, or scrotum. Week two, the massage can include breast touch. Week three, breasts and butt touch is allowed. Week four, breasts, butt, vulva, and scrotum touch are allowed, but with no digital penetration. Week five, massaging breasts, butt, vulva, labia, clitoris, scrotum, and penis are allowed, but still with no penetration or stroking to orgasm. You get the picture! Your tantric journey should culminate in the sexual experience that allows you to feel most connected. For some people, that's oral sex, for others it's penetrative sex, while for others it might be something else entirely.

1.   Invite your partner into a space that feels not only safe and comfortable but also sexy (use your sexual template work!). You can use a timer or trust your intuition.

2.   Either naked or clothed in non-constricting clothes, sit facing each other.

3.   Put your right hand on your heart and hold left hands.

4.   Look into each other's eyes, which in tantra is called "eye-gazing," and hold for thirty seconds to a minute. (Feel free to blink—it's not a

staring contest; it's about being present.) Also, if you notice your eyes darting back and forth, look at your partner's left eye, so you're gazing left eye to left eye. It's natural to laugh or feel uncomfortable in the early weeks, but stick with it. Eye-gazing is a direct route to increased empathy and intimacy (into me, see).

5. Release hands, then give an appreciation for your partner's willingness, such as, "I appreciate that you took time out of your schedule to prioritize our sex life," or "I appreciate that you're always up for something new with me."

6. Decide who is going to give first and who will receive first.

7. For seven to eight minutes, the giver will give the receiver a massage. (I'm particular about seven to eight minutes because nine to ten minutes is often too relaxing, reducing the potential for erotic energy.) The receiver can make constructive and affirming comments about pressure, speed, and the areas they like massaged most and least. Avoid negative comments unless something hurts, in which case, be sure to speak up. This is not a dialogue. The giver should simply listen.

8. Switch roles and perform a seven- to eight-minute massage.

9. Come back together and sit facing each other. This time hold both of your partner's hands, and eye-gaze for thirty seconds to a minute.

10. Offer an appreciation for the pleasure and, if you felt it, the connection. Say something like, "Thank you for helping me feel in touch with my body," or "I appreciate how connected you felt to me."

Reflections on the Weave

What are you giving more of?

What are you getting more of?

How do you feel more connected to your partner?

In what ways does your connection feel different?

- Are there any ways that connection is still challenging? If so, how?

The weave of tantra combined with the progressive structure of sensate focus creates a safe container for healing and passion.[121] Knowing where you're going builds safety, while open communication offers sexual agency, and anticipation generates desire as you and your partner are left wanting more as the weeks evolve. Talk about your "homework" throughout the week. Bring it up in casual conversation when your partner isn't rushed or stressed, or try sending a sext about what you're imagining the two of you will do. Your homework will build a healthy habit of connection that you'll long for, as well as miss in its absence.

Sexual trauma diminished your ability to authentically connect with yourself, others, the present moment, and your eroticism. Every step you take toward reconnection replenishes your faith in your choices as responses to what you want rather than reactions to what you've feared. Your body and its inherent discernment is an essential gauge for reassessing how you connect and whom you connect with. Trust your gut. From there, lean on your presence and awareness, which is neither anxious nor numb. Celebrate how far you've come, your indisputable resiliency and willingness to rediscover the gifts of connection. Embrace your thriver spirit. Your body offers guidance while your soul offers expansion. There's no limitation on connection. As poet Della Hicks Wilson writes, "Your soul doesn't have bones for a reason."[122]

Take a deep breath. Give yourself a hug. You have made it beautifully and powerfully through the foundation of your sexual reclamation. With your newfound insights and applications of control, pleasure, and connection, you're set to pursue and delight in a restored and reenergized sex life. You have everything you need. You're whole. Keep practicing with yourself and others. Chapter 10, the last full chapter of the book, serves as an extension to your foundation—a patio, of sorts, on your well-constructed home—that you can step onto and off of as you desire. It offers a space of sexual reimagining through fantasy. What you learn may feel essential in rewriting your thriver story, or it may simply be of interest from a place of curiosity. Both stances are stellar—you're already golden. Chapter 10 is yet another offering and choice on your path to passion.

CHAPTER TEN

Sex Reimagined

*Our erotic knowledge empowers us, becomes a lens through which
we scrutinize all aspects of our existence, forcing us to evaluate those
aspects honestly in terms of their relative meaning within our lives.
And this is a grave responsibility, projected from within each of us,
not to settle for the convenient, the shoddy, the conventionally
expected, nor the merely safe.*

—Audre Lorde

By now you know that sex worth wanting is much more than a genital-based encounter. Sex has the capacity to be an expansive mind-body experience where the power of intimacy allows freedom from fear and sheer aliveness. What's left in your journey, should you want more, is the subtle yet exquisite facet of sex that makes it erotic. By settling even more deeply into spaciousness rather than constriction, you can play with the reformulation of your sexual identity; in this situation, your trauma is a part of your sexual story but no longer its entirety. From this position, you will sit solidly in knowing what you lost and what you gained, what you're ready to give away, and what you must reclaim. This is your personal erotic resurrection.

As you continue the process of learning to trust your mind and body, you're poised to look beyond what's necessary into what's possible. Your natural creativity paired with sexual curiosity nudges you to ask,

"What's next?" The answer? *Fantasy*, the art of sex. In this last instructive chapter, you'll learn to use your erotic imagination to let go of limiting beliefs and prescribed roles relegated by your trauma. Sex will be sexy again—not an obligation, not a trigger, but a gateway to desire.

Story: *Playfully Yours*

Hannah and Nathan looked like they'd just stepped out of a glossy magazine. She had a boho-chic vibe, too perfectly thrown together to be thrown together at all. Nathan evinced a pitch-perfect corporate guy look, his tailored suit and shined shoes letting me know control was high on his list of needs. I could also tell he didn't want to be here. Of course, Hannah knew too and quickly jumped in to save him. "We're here because of me," she announced. "I can't handle intimacy and it's ruining our life."

"Wow, that's a big statement," I replied. "Thank you for being so accountable and brave, I might add. But I have yet to meet a couple where the problem belongs entirely to one partner. Relationships, by nature, are dynamic."

Nathan sat silently as Hannah hurriedly relayed her history. She said she wanted to get through it so we could address the "real problem." She explained that her parents divorced when she was two and neither offered much supervision during her preteen years. She started drinking and doing drugs, and ended up working at strip clubs in her late teens and early twenties. She said she had only ever had sex drunk or high. Her boyfriend before Nathan was emotionally and physically abusive, and he'd often had sex with her when she didn't want to. At this point she took a deep breath and said, "He's a complete monster, I know that, but I think I kind of liked the abuse. I mean not the hitting, but our rough sex."

"No one likes abuse and especially not rape, but a lot of people like rough sex," I responded. "I have a feeling there was something in those experiences that made you feel more in control or empowered, even just for a moment."

Hannah frustratedly added, "I don't even care anymore. I don't want to think about that life ever again. And I want it out of our relationship. I'm so angry!"

She sat back and put her head in her hands. I asked Nathan what he was feeling. "I feel she's right," he curtly offered. "It's not working. What she needs I can't do. I love her, but I won't be treated this way."

I asked Nathan to say more, and he finally offered his interpretation of the problem. Hannah needed sex to include choking and spanking for her to orgasm, and he wasn't into it. He said, "I tried it and I just can't do that to her. She tries to do it to me sometimes, and I really hate that."

Hannah started to cry and kept repeating, "I'm sorry. I'm so sorry." Nathan hugged her, which couples who are angry don't often do without prompting. Witnessing this, I knew there was plenty of love and forgiveness left to give in this relationship.

Hannah, Nathan, and I worked together for the next eight months, slowly pulling apart what felt abusive or compulsive, and what was a preference versus what was a fantasy. They approached the sessions from a place of curiosity and creativity to imagine how preference and fantasy could coexist in the loving and passionate relationship they were coauthoring. After completing numerous weeks of sensate focus and tantra exercises to ground them in connection (chapter 9), I created weekly homework exercises that included a slow, methodical sharing of their sexual preferences and fantasies. These were never demands, but rather offerings. There was always plenty of communication before they *"played" (the word they preferred to "homework"), as well as affirmations and reassuring body language during and eye-gazing afterward. They are still experimenting, particularly with fantasy, but as things stand now, choking is completely off their erotic menu but spanking is sometimes on it. Its meaning was transformed from shameful to playful. They are now reimagining what they want their relational eroticism to embody, free of the past.*

Story Reflections

In your journal, reflect on how you relate to Hannah and Nathan's story.

Did their previous dynamic feel familiar at all? If yes, how so?

How are sexual preferences or fantasies pushing you and your partner apart, or are they the glue holding you together?

What do you think introducing healthy fantasy into your sexual relationships will feel like?

What are your concerns around sharing your fantasies with your partner?

What are two ways you would like to see more playfulness in your sexual relationship, and how would that change things for the better?

How do you imagine your relationships will thrive when your fantasies are no longer attached to shame?

The Body Erotic

When it comes to the difference between sex and eroticism, one of my favorite descriptions comes from Finn Deerhart, a sex and intimacy coach who works mainly with gay and queer men. He says, "Sex is a function of body parts; eroticism is a cultivated art."[123] Like art, eroticism confers subjectivity and mystery—it arouses meaning. Eroticism inter-laced with sex is a thoughtfully curated experience. When you find your-self in an erotic space rather than a purely sexual one, you'll notice a charged intensity as well as the propensity to play and a capacity for otherness. The enigmatic essence of eroticism allows you to try on differ-ent sexual personas. It's about exploration, not an end point; there's no performance-related goal. You are not a person having sex but a person being sex—the duality of self and sex should be long gone.

Thus far, your path from surviving to thriving had to be rooted in the present, necessarily stepping away from the hurts of the past as well as worry about the future. But, as you begin to navigate within the more relaxed boundaries of sexual and relational health, you can escape into a mental and physical expanse that isn't fixed in time, place, or charac-ter, but morphs intuitively. In the erotic, you can be bonded or autono-mous, fantastical or literal, implausible or entirely possible. With safety and trust as givens, risk and expansion are yours to explore. Like your overall process of thriving, your relationships must exude a life force of their own. Your relationships live in service to your *self*. With that in mind, there's one foundational principle of eroticism that you must pursue with complete and utter persistence: don't deny your truth in the presence of intimacy. You've tried denying it. It doesn't work. Hiding your pain only makes it fight harder to be seen, and disowning it only means it owns you. Your partner and the passionate world you're creating are opportunities to rewrite your erotic story, one where your past still exists but amplifies your ability to see and be seen.

Cultivating fantasy within the erotic offers a chance to flirt, play, and even pretend. Like many survivors, perhaps you haven't explored fantasy because you haven't felt safe. That makes sense, and it also doesn't make you strange for fantasizing, or incapable of fantasizing. Remember, anxiety overrides cognition, and if you couldn't think prop-erly, you certainly couldn't fantasize without dissociating or panicking. Like good sex, fantasizing is a practice. You are not showing up late to the game. Conversely, you have a keen awareness of the entire field and rules of play, namely consent and pleasure.

Regarding the former, you may worry that consent isn't sexy. That's untrue. Only with a baseline of consent can sex be sexy; to say otherwise denies your truth. Your authenticity allows fantasy to serve as a useful tool for cultivating passion. In my opinion, believing that consent isn't sexy should be excised from societal expectations, along with the idea that only if unwanted sex is violent is it actually bad enough to be traumatic! This is an ongoing issue. In her book about rethinking women's desire and lust, *Untrue*, writer and cultural critic Wednesday Martin points to too much "hand-wringing" on the part of people who falsely believe that movements like #MeToo and #TimesUp are robbing women of desire and agency, "complaining that consent is unromantic and will be the death of flirtation."[124] As you venture into fantasy, know that the exact opposite is true—consent precedes pleasure, and pleasure precedes passion. Again, consent *is* sexy.

Have you dared to engage with your sexual fantasies? Have they scared or excited you, or perhaps both? Do you understand what you fantasize about? If you answered "yes," "maybe," or even "no," you are in the land of eroticism. If you thought to yourself, "But I don't fantasize," I guarantee you actually do. Whether your fantasy is as tame as your partner telling you that you look beautiful, or as taboo as a stranger ripping your clothes off and having sex with you in a public place, both fantasies translate to feeling empowered, desirable, and unmistakably wanted. If you fantasize about getting away from family, friends, work, and all of your devices, or about completely submitting to your hot boss, both fantasies impart your desire to abdicate responsibility and decision making. Understanding your fantasies is yet another way to reduce shame and reveal pleasure. Whether you're in a long-term monogamous relationship or single and ready to date, fantasies impart meaning to what you want to *feel* more so than what you actually want to *do*.

Remember, eroticism is about meaning—the *art* of sex, not the *act* of sex. When you find meaning, you'll also find passion.

Here's your opportunity to reconsider your fantasies without immediately denying, rejecting, or hiding them. In her work with clients around sexual fantasy, sex therapist Nazanin Moali notes that repressing fantasies doesn't make them go away but instead simply lets them remain undealt with. As she explains, "It's much more fun to explore your sexuality with a trusted partner than to deny that it exists and perpetuate a shame cycle."[125] Thus, while you're being careful to not deny your truth, please don't deny yourself permission to explore. While each of us to a certain extent ascribes to the social and cultural fantasies we've grown up with, it's critical not to buy into them without sexual self-awareness. You can't entirely remove the lens of your upbringing or your trauma (you are the lens!), but you can widen it. In other words, if you fantasize about something you think you shouldn't, get curious rather than judgmental. Repression or rejection are founded either in fear or shame, or most likely both. Similar to how you used to repress the truth of your sexual trauma—and your body, emotions, relationships, or sexuality had to bear the suffering—repressing your sexual fantasies prolongs internalized shame. Like your trauma, your fantasies are a part of you, but they certainly don't define you. They are almost never a literal translation of intent, but rather an abstract expression of significance. For example, if you're into dad-bod guys rather than beefcakes, ask yourself what that might mean. Is it about feeling safer? Or perhaps it's about feeling more accepted or acceptable, or even more powerful? Or could it be about rebuking societal norms, puritanical culture, and capitalism? If you can fantasize without judgment, you're a step closer to Eros—vitality, freedom, and sexual irrepressibility.

Remember, your fantasies are your own making, born of your beautifully seductive and provocative imagination. They aren't meant to scare you. At best, they are a mind-body offering, another item on the menu.

What you imagine is not what you have to do. You can try it and not like it. You can try it and love it and want to do it again. Or you can try it and be on the fence, neither a solid yes nor a definitive no. Your fantasy life can equate to your "real" life, but more often than not it simply—though importantly—informs it. The fantasy is the fire; what you do with the burn is totally up to you. When considering the paradox of what you fanaticize about versus what you want to act out, sex therapist and author Ian Kerner offers this: "The sex we have in our lives—familiar, repetitious—is usually very different from the sex we have in our fantasies—exaggerated, taboo—and perhaps that's the point."[126]

When it comes to exploring fantasies, the influence of novelty and taboo cannot be overstated. As humans, we love to break free from the tried and true, and sometimes even be naughty doing so. There aren't many places in our lives where we get to be bad or (heaven forbid!) shameless. For the most part, we toe the line.

I find this is especially true of survivors. Because maintaining a sense of control is so crucial for survivors to feel safe while they move through the world, the naughtiness of fantasy isn't typically an option. It's easy to confuse excitement with danger, and then err on the side of caution. But let me reassure you that fantasies are by their nature safe—and therefore consensual—because they are happening in your head! You *are* in control. Like the sex you're having, if your fantasy is consensual and pleasurable, it's good. Here's yet another opportunity to let yourself off the hook!

Understanding your sexual fantasies—their meaning, significance, and viability—is an integral part of your healthy sexuality and erotic empowerment. The following list offers some of the most common fantasies, but for a deeper dive into sexual fantasies and their meanings, check out sexuality researcher Justin Lehmiller's book, *Tell Me What You Want: The Science of Sexual Desire and How It Can Help You Improve Your Sex Life.*[127]

Common Sexual Fantasies

Dirty talk

Threesomes or multiple partner sex

Same sex/queer sex

Rough sex/BDSM (bondage/domination/sadism/masochism)

Voyeurism

Exhibitionism

Public sex

Novel positions (cowgirl, doggy style, spooning, standing, etc.)

Toys (vibrators, dildos, butt plugs, etc.)

Props (handcuffs, feathers, candles, swings, cushions, food, ice, etc.)

Role-play

Pornography (creating it, being in it, or engaging with it)

Fetishes (feet, lingerie, pantyhose, leather, latex, gloves, boots, etc.)

Common Sexual Fantasies Reflections

After reading the list, what are you feeling? For example, shock, comfort, curiosity, or acceptance?

How does that internal feeling match your external expression of your sexuality?

What meaning do you make from the fantasies that resonate with you?

Think bigger than these acts of sex—what themes may need more attention in your life, such as power, selfishness, taking risks, self-actualization, or novelty?

Eroticism in Action

Recognizing your fantasies and ascribing meaning to them is one thing, and sharing them is quite another. Like the story of your sexual trauma, you never have to share your fantasies unless you want to. It's not the details that matter, only that you are free of shame in asking for what you want. Your truth has boundaries. Know them, no matter whether you're talking about something bad that happened or something good that might happen. Honor your limits, but also allow yourself some flexibility (that's Eros).

Boundaries aren't always a locked cage. They can be a set of malleable convictions that shift, at your will, depending on the time, situation, and other people involved. What is a hard boundary with your new romantic interest may not be a boundary at all with your trusted long-term partner. Or it might be. This is where the somatic element of your journey to thriving shines. Trust your gut, and more important, trust yourself. Again, you have control. Maintain and relinquish it based on your current desires, not your past worries.

If you decide to share your fantasy, ask yourself some questions first. Is the information a call to action, an intention for a later date, fuel for the relationship's erotic fire, or simply the conveyance of a quality you want more of, like power, control, objectification, submission, or recklessness? Knowing what you want from your fantasy—even your best guess in the moment—is essential. Eros, your life force, is by nature unrestrained and a risk-taker, but can only thrive within a space of genuineness and safety. In *Getting the Sex You Want*, sex therapist Tammy Nelson points to the importance of well-informed intention around fantasy. She writes, "What we choose to take from fantasy to action should be determined by our personal boundaries and a sense of integrity."[128] Unlike your sexual trauma, where your body and emotions were misused without your consent, when it comes to your fantasies, you get to decide what to share and what to hold sacred.

Let's pause. Take a breath and imagine, whether or not you have a current partner, what sharing a sexual fantasy might feel like. Yes, you can expect it to feel a little scary (remember, a central facet of Eros is unpredictability), but it should also feel empowering, like another solid step into relational health and sexual selfhood. If the goals of sharing are to continue to free yourself from sexual shame, elevate what you know about yourself as a sexual being, practice asking for what you want, and increase passion in your relationships, you're as close to ready as you can be. From here, your work is to turn your expanded sexual consciousness into an impassioned, transparent endeavor, letting your partner into your previously secretive world. Sharing your sexual fantasies and the meaning they confer is a spark to your relational fire in and of itself. Stepping into Eros and fantasy naturally transcends self and embraces other. As therapist Esther Perel notes, "Sex becomes both a way to illuminate conflicts over intimacy and desire, and a way to begin to heal these destructive splits."[129]

How does this process work? We'll get to the logistics in a moment, but the overall premise is this. When you share the innermost workings of your erotic imagination, it creates differentiation between you and your partner, which fuels desire. It lets your partner know, "Oh, I don't know everything about you!" Novelty is the seat of human desire, and by presenting a formerly uncharted part of yourself, there is not only a new story to tell but also a new you to reveal. This resurrection is vital for you to feel and equally important for your partner to understand. You are so much more than a survivor. Not only are you not broken, but you're also not fragile. You can own your sexual needs and desires. Sexual agency and fantasy go in hand in hand.

As far as the actual sharing is concerned, there are several ways to go about it. The first is spontaneously. Choose a moment when you and your partner are feeling present, unencumbered with work or other stressors, and most importantly, connected. However, I do not recommend sharing immediately before having sex, while having sex, or right after having sex. Similar to the exercises around connection in chapter 9, use these discussions to plan for passionate sex and build anticipation. Sharing before or during sex puts too much pressure to perform on yourself and your partner. Another option comes from therapist and author Angelika Eck, who created an exercise that entails you and your partner each writing one sexual fantasy on a piece of paper and putting it in a sealed envelope. Before you share, she suggests asking yourself these questions: Do you want your partner to see it? How do you know? What are the possible benefits? What are some potential downsides? From there, you can decide whether or not to share.[130]

There are many other exercises you can try to share fantasies in a healthy way. Psychologist Michael Bader's book, *Arousal*, is a great resource to utilize. In my work with survivors, the following exercise has been especially effective in helping both partners feel secure yet adventurous within the connected dynamic of the relationship.

Sharing Fantasies

This exercise should occur at an agreed-upon time and place in order to give both you and your partner ample time to prepare. It can be done clothed or naked, in a tone that is lighthearted and simply meant to communicate curiosity, or in a more serious manner that creates a seductive tenor. For either mood, utilizing Kegels helps to deepen the awareness of your sexual body. In case Kegels are new to you, they are repetitive movements by which you contract and relax the muscles in your pelvic floor, as if you were trying to voluntarily stop urinating and then start again. This strengthens your pelvic floor, but not just for bladder control. Kegels improve numerous aspects of sexual functioning, including the ability to have stronger orgasms, and people of every gender and bodily configuration can do them. Their purpose within the context of this exercise is to connect a bodily, somatic element to your erotic imagination.

1. Sit facing each other holding hands, and maintain eye contact.

2. Breathe in and out slowly, and try to co-regulate your breath with your partner's.

3. On the in breath, do a Kegel and squeeze your pelvic floor.

4. On the out breath, release the Kegel and feel your pelvic floor relax (repeat the in and out breaths three times).

5. Share one element of your sexual fantasy as concisely as possible.

6. Your partner will reflect your fantasy by saying something like, "I understand that you are curious about _____. Is that correct?"

7. You answer "Yes" or "Not exactly," and restate your fantasy.

8. Your partner shares one element of their fantasy.

9. You reflect their fantasy by saying something like, "I understand that you are curious about _____. Is that correct?"

10. They answer "Yes" or "Not exactly," and restate their fantasy.

11. Offer each other an appreciation for sharing, like "I appreciate that you shared that part of yourself because _____."

Take the next five minutes to discuss whether the fantasy is something you would like to bring into your sex life immediately, or whether for now you'd prefer to watch it or read about it together. Or, you can decide you'd like the fantasy to remain a fantasy, and simply enjoy the deeper erotic understanding and connection it is engendering in your relationship.

Exercise Reflections

In your journal, reflect on your experience of the fantasy sharing exercise.

What did you feel when you shared? Were you nervous, excited, shy, or emboldened, for example?

How did you feel when your partner reflected your fantasy?

What did you feel when your partner shared their fantasy? Were you anxious, curious, or judgmental, for example?

In what ways can you understand more about your partner's erotic world without making it about you—namely, not taking it as something you're lacking or not doing right?

How was your partner able to understand your erotic world without making it about them?

In what ways did this help create sexual intensity?

Name one way you find your partner sexier.

Name one way you find yourself sexier.

Indulging your erotic creativity not only offers the opportunity to learn more about yourself, but it also challenges you to reimagine sex as a cocreated, exciting experience. Passion lives in emotional regulation and bodily collaboration, and it finds its ideal balance in the sometimes messy but always vital space between probability and possibility. Your willingness to consider—and potentially share—your innermost fantasies is a testament to your resiliency. Your sexuality cannot be minimized or marginalized solely by an act, whether it was painful (your trauma) or is arousing (your fantasies). Those insular days of feeling bad about the sex you had, are having, or want to have can take their deserved place in your past.

As you continue to thrive, you'll notice that you have an abundance of choice around sex. Whether you're engaged in your self-pleasure practice or in a dance of intimacy with a partner, the opportunities for mind-body connection are endless. Your reimagined sex life can include flirtation, sexting, kissing, penetration, role-play, and fantasizing—or none of these! You never again have to do anything or feel anything in the sacred space of your sexuality that you don't choose to. You have what you need to create the sexual and relational life you want. You can lean on control, pleasure, and connection to feel safe, understood, and appreciated, and tread determinedly into fantasy to feel a bit wild, or even radical, in the best possible way. Your boundaries are solid and your sexual agency is well honed. Rather than holding on for dear life as you've had to in the past, you can let go and escape into an erotic world of your making.

You have taken care of yourself. Thank you for picking up this book, for letting your body speak its mind, for letting yourself off the hook, and for tending to your pleasure and passion. Your hard-won progress earned by looking inward can finally rest. Not only do you deserve it, but you also need it. Believe it or not, there is such a thing as too much introspection. Numerous studies have shown that the happiest people hold a healthy sense of proportion of self-focus and the bigger picture of the world.[131] If you're anything like the majority of my clients, taking a break from yourself will come as a welcome relief. Your work in this moment is to sharpen your external lens, your sensitive, empathetic gaze outward. This won't diminish your story; it will amplify it, perfectly in chorus with others. Not only does the load of suffering become lighter in its sharing, but the sharing also heals—you, them, all of us. The final chapter manifests your collective voice, how your healing is *the* healing and the change the world has been waiting for.

Thriving as Your Social Declaration

I will use Brock's name, but the truth is he could be Brad or Brody or Benson, and it doesn't matter. The point is not their individual significance, but their commonality, all the people enabling a broken system...I want to leave them behind so I can move forward.

—Chanel Miller

Can you say it, out loud, one more time? *"That was then, this is now."* And it goes deeper. That was surviving, this is thriving. Surviving was then, thriving is now. Surviving was getting through your days, thriving is enjoying them. You will always be a survivor as a way of acknowledging the sexual trauma you've endured, but you are a thriver in how you live, love, and embrace what's next. It is only through thriving that you can usher in a future full of self-acceptance, solid relationships, and great sex. Your emotions are yours to own, your body yours to inhabit, your relationships yours to welcome, and your sexuality yours to reclaim.

Thriving is a deeply personal process indeed, but it is one that is unequivocally strengthened by collective consciousness. Thank you for no longer denying or minimizing your trauma. Thank you for being one of millions to leave the secret parts of yourself behind in order to recover what you've lost, to claim what is rightfully yours. This is both the arduous and the joyous time when you settle into your tried and tested resilience and begin to reimagine who you are in the world. You are not damaged or unrelatable or untouchable or unsexy or unlovable. There are too many of you, too many of us, for that to be true.

I want you to understand that the brokenness you felt because of your sexual trauma is actually a brokenness in ideology. You are normal. Having to survive sexual trauma is not. What's more, the systems we have to deal with sexual trauma are entirely deficient. We've done this work so that you can transcend that system and create a new reality that is focused on you, your pleasure, your safety, and your eroticism. So please, don't forsake yourself to spare a deficient system. The system can go screw itself.

With that said, what then is the final frontier of transforming a personal resurrection into a social declaration? It seems only fitting to ask for three intentions as a powerful accompaniment to your three-part process (control, pleasure, and connection) of thriving.

1. Retell Your Story. Telling your story is an essential act of dissent. Staying silent only serves perpetrators by keeping things as they are, not as they should be. While most survivors benefit from telling their story and experiencing a sense of collective compassion, it isn't sharing details of your traumatic experience that's ultimately most healing. You never have to tell anyone—not your friends, family, partner, or even your therapist—the specifics of what happened to you, but you do have to tell the story differently to yourself. You must change your relationship to your story; you must hear it differently in your head and feel it differently in your body.

In this version, you are in control of the most important thing possible—not what happened, but how you feel about what happened; namely, how you feel about yourself. Retell your story in a way that places blame where it belongs, freeing you of emotional and physical pain by freeing you of culpability. Retell it in a way that once and for all lets you off the hook. This is the chapter in your story where you never again take responsibility for your perpetrator's bad behavior, offenses, or crimes. To be unapologetically blunt, you didn't rape, abuse, assault, or harass yourself. It's your turn to be unapologetic and unabashed, to shout aloud the sheer absurdity of survivor shame.

Retelling your story by telling the truth is certainly scary, but ultimately, it is less scary than being in pain or endlessly running from it. When you give your emotions, body, sexuality, and relationships a voice, you give them choice. Choice is your antidote to fear. Sexual trauma took away your choice, but retelling gives it back. You are the protagonist now, the lead actor in your movie—the thriver, supporter, torchbearer, champion, and spokesperson for change. How you change and how you support that change is entirely up to you. It can be quietly personal or deliberately public. You can break the systemic cycle of violence by living in a healthier body, a body free from pain and shame. You can erode the disinformation by claiming the loving relationships you deserve. You can dismantle untruths by helping another survivor more clearly see their truth. You can subvert shame by volunteering at a rape crisis center and telling your family and friends about it. You can destabilize a flawed belief system by proclaiming your thrivership communally, whether a podcast for thousands, a presentation for hundreds, or a small address at your local high school. Or you can dethrone the holders and abusers of sexual power by calling them out and pointing a finger that will eventually elicit shame from its rightful source.

And you can report. This is your right and another choice. Reporting a sexual offense to authorities helps retell your story in two ways. The first is for you, as you have an opportunity to reclaim your power in a court of law. The second is for all survivors, as we get to reclaim our power in the court of public opinion. The old story that false reporting is a significant problem regarding sexual offenses is erroneous at best, crippling at worst. It is categorically *not* a problem and certainly not a significant one. Survivors do not frequently make false reports, as the sex-negative and survivor-blaming system would like you to believe. Sexual offenses are falsely reported at exactly the same rate as other felonies, between 2 and 8 percent.[132] If your retelling includes reporting, do so with this fact in hand. You believe yourself, finally, and other survivors believe you too. The final undertaking is your persistent optimism that one day all survivors will be believed.

Your old story was not a reflection of your true self, but the loss of it.[133] You were not your trauma, but rather an amalgamation of its effects. Your retold story is one of self-forgiveness—the ultimate gift—resilience and evolution. History, herstory, and theirstory is written, and while there's no changing what was, there is changing what can be. The present moment, free of fear, will reframe your healing. Feeling safe will allow you to finally feel well. As author and sexual healer David Wichman wrote in his own story of surviving abuse and assault, "This story is not happening in me any longer; it's happening through me. I stand with it and carry it as my light. I believe we are all messengers, and we have come to share a message that brings us closer to love and closer to kindness as a way of life, where kindness becomes our first response instead of a reaction born of fear and self-protection."[134]

2. Dare to Empathize. Can you imagine using empathy rather than fear as your navigator? What if you step into vulnerability rather than shoring up your defenses? Often, it's the empathetic gaze that can give us our clearest reflections. I am decidedly not a believer in the idiom, "You can't love others until you learn to love yourself." Sometimes it's your proficiency for giving that ultimately opens to receiving—when you offer acceptance and nurturing, you in turn learn what genuine acceptance and nurturance feels like.

You likely have years of practice denying the truth of your trauma and living in shame, so it makes sense that you might also deny the truth of love. Shame is a direct barrier to love. Yet, by nature of your survivorship, you are highly sensitive and acutely attuned, thus expressing sympathy for others is a well-honed skill. You likely felt it for the survivors portrayed in this book, and you've likely felt it in the lived stories swirling around you, whether explicitly spoken or silently sustained. Back then, you probably compared experiences of suffering. You likely told yourself what other people suffered through was worse than your own suffering, which let you feel deeply for them but less so, or not at all, for yourself. I hope that one thing that's been made clear through our work together is that you can't measure suffering—all suffering is suffering. It's all "bad enough." Sympathy was your way in, but empathy is unquestionably your way out. Having empathy for the collective survivor experience highlights the power and grace of mutuality. Actor, survivor, and sexual justice activist Michaela Coel, who also plays a survivor in HBO's series *I May Destroy You*, says the act of empathy helped her move forward as an artist and a person. She believes empathy, at its core, is about her own well-being. "This makes *me* feel better," she explains. "It's about how you can feel better in a system that is fucked, but you need to sleep well. Daring to empathize, daring to help other people as well as being helped, it will do *you* good. It's about *you*."[135]

One of your most powerful acts moving forward is communicating empathy through solidarity. That aloneness you felt in your experience of surviving was entirely untrue. You've never been alone. The #MeToo movement shone a stark light on this reality. It was and is a momentous declaration for survivors to share their stories, use their voices, commune in their collective power, and demand retribution and change. In 2017, #MeToo[136] and its partner movement #TimesUp[137] went viral, giving the world a wake-up call to the magnitude of sexual misconduct and its destructive, often lifelong effects. These movements were the catalyst for change so many survivors had been waiting for, whether consciously or not. By reading this book and sharing its message, you're doing personally what #MeToo and #TimesUp did globally. You're voicing your truth, which is *the* truth, validating suffering, and placing blame where it belongs. Like thriving, collective healing takes risk. It might be easier to remain quiet, continue to play nice, and not cause a stir. But "easy" isn't what the broken system gave you, so it's definitely not what you have to give back. If you need any more permission, here it is: make a scene!

Vulnerable, empathetic sharing will not always feel good, but inevitably, in the long race toward change, it is the path of least resistance. Your body won't have to shout anymore. Don't forget that when you heal the trauma, you heal the body, and when you heal the body, you heal the mind. From there, solid friendships, healthy intimate relationships, and good sex follow. However, daring to empathize is not a promise of perfection or a waveless trajectory from feeling bad to feeling good; it's a call to practice. Other than love, there is no action that so obviously blossoms in reciprocity. When you feel bad, reach out instead of retreating in. Feel for others, which will instinctively help you feel for yourself. Let your allies—the people who believe you and respect you—be sounding boards for your conquests and your foibles. Promise yourself to never again deny empathy by concealing your authenticity. Perhaps daring to empathize equates to staying tender, as survivor and author Chanel Miller suggests: "Stay tender with your power. Never fight to injure, fight to uplift. Fight because you know that in this life you deserve safety, joy, and freedom."[138] Your empathy and tenderness for every survivor will ultimately dismantle a system that operates on its denial.

3. Have Great Sex. If retelling your story is an essential act of dissent, having great sex is the ultimate expression of it. What could further derail a system than to brazenly pursue the power it intended to suppress? There's nothing more dangerous to society's passive acceptance of sexual misconduct than your sexual empowerment. Having great sex is your legacy. When you feel sexy, you feel entitled to pleasure and righteous in asking for it; once you've held the gratification that's legitimately yours, you certainly don't have to hand it back.

No matter what your version of great sex looks like, each encounter frees decades upon decades of repression. Sex as weapon and sex as healer are fundamentally incompatible bedfellows. Bad sex almost always equates to shameful sex. As we've discussed, when you felt shame, you lost the agency to feel anything else. Great sex, on the other hand, is shameless! It includes a chorus of feelings, from lustful and confident to playful or even demure. Having great sex is the definitive proclamation that your body's sovereignty is restored. Your pleasure is an essential part of building the sex-positive world everyone you know deserves, whether your blood family, family of choice, or your descendants many years from now. Your ability to reclaim pleasure inherently brings humankind along with you and will help change the future.

Having great sex also reminds you to drop the story that to be loved, you must pretend. You can't pretend to have great sex any more than you can continue to pretend you're fine with feeling unsafe, disrespected, and disempowered. You might fool your partner, but you can't fool yourself! Pretending in the bedroom is a performance; the exclamation of a fake orgasm only perpetuates the cycle of settling for less. Moreover, pretending in *any* aspect of life robs others of the experience of truly knowing you. You can't sit in empathy if you're still sitting in inauthenticity. Having great sex will at long last dissuade you from the belief that when you're "over" this, you'll be worthy of a loving relationship. There's no "over." There's no lightning bolt moment of thriving. There's only the deliberate chiseling away at the barriers to control, pleasure, and connection. Having great sex will teach you the exact opposite of what trauma taught you about sex. Rather than making you feel deficient, dissociated, or rejected, you'll feel competent, present, and prioritized.

It may sound overambitious to suggest your choice to have great sex can change the world, but honestly, it's not that far of a stretch. If the sex you have from this moment forward is framed in sex positivity—again, the concept that all sex is good sex as long as it's consensual and pleasurable—you are structurally weakening cultural acceptance of nonconsensual, unpleasurable sex. There is no pleasure without consent, so it makes sense this is where sexual rights activists are striking the first chord.

Since #MeToo, many of our conversations around sexuality are reexamining consent and what is considered outside its lines. For example, "rape by fraud" is a construct that questions the level to which duplicity constitutes a lack of consent. As of right now, when someone deceives a person to get them into bed, it is not illegal. However, activists are pushing for a law stipulating that anyone who lies or withholds information about something that would be a deal breaker—anything that would have changed your mind about sleeping with them—equates to a lack of consent and thus is sexual misconduct. Effectively, if you had known the truth, you never would have consented to sex. Thus, there was no consent, and sex without consent is assault.[139]

The nuance of illegality is important, of course. Lying isn't a crime, but when the lie impacts the sovereignty of the body, it offers pause for thought. And though we are no longer seeing #MeToo or #TimesUp constantly trending, we can be certain, and thankful, the conversation isn't going away. In just the last two years there's been a marked change, as more survivors speak out and more perpetrators are brought to justice. It's become culturally unacceptable to let abuse slip through the cracks, which is a huge and necessary shift in ideology.

As a survivor, you've been forced to challenge what is acceptable and unacceptable in your sexual experiences. You've had to carefully self-examine those moments you gave someone the benefit of the doubt and perhaps shouldn't have, when you "let things slide" that should have stopped. It is time for a total upheaval of our expectations around good sex. This will, at first, naturally hold us in ambiguity, but eventually establish a new standard of acceptability. As physician, addiction therapist, and author Gabor Maté suggests, "No society can fully understand itself without looking at its shadow side."[140] Consent is the survivor culture's shadow side; looking deeply is our triumph.

Pain was your way into healing, but pleasure is your way out. Your willingness to think and feel differently about your sexual trauma, and in some ways reexperience it, is awe worthy. Thank you for picking up this book and reconnecting with desire. Thank you for wanting more, and most importantly, thank you for being unwilling to settle for less.

Perhaps now you can acutely feel how victimhood is a role and survivorship is a state, but thrivership is your well-deserved way of life. Yet, no matter how much health you've recovered or strength you've regained, there is nothing I can offer that will ever make your suffering worth it. There is no parity between suffering and growth, no scale that tips to finally make this all feel fair. Like forgiveness, fairness isn't the goal. The goal is reclaiming pleasure and passion in a way that frees your mind and body of judgment, that lets it rest in its own unique remarkability. And remember, collective healing is *the* force for societal change. Your process of reclamation may look entirely dissimilar to another survivor's. That's okay! Their suffering is not your suffering, their process is not your process, but their healing is your healing and yours, theirs. The goal is not to be the same, only to go together toward a place of healing.

In this moment your thrivership is holding you up with millions of others. With this knowledge, I hope you can fully realize your strength in spite of your suffering. Your trauma has taken a lot, and my wish is that in your reclamation, you've gained a fair amount, too. In contrast to surviving, thriving gives you more awareness, more truth, more pride for all you've overcome, and certainly more pleasure wherever you can discover it.

Your trauma history was never meant to inform your life; connection, intimacy, and Eros, your vital life force, were. On the days when you feel like you aren't living big enough or working hard enough, you're doing perfectly. The simple intent of integration—peace and ease between your mind and body—feels like inaction, but it's very much the opposite. You're finally able to let yourself be rather than pushing yourself to survive. Remember, pleasure is your nonnegotiable prerequisite for living, your infinitely reclaimable resource. Some days it will feel like fireworks, especially if you're having great sex. Other days, pleasure will seem intangible. Listen. Listen to your body, listen to your feelings, listen to the global refrain of voices that are whispering, pleading, and demanding a revolution. Continue to withdraw your silence as a way to withdraw the system's shame-based currency. Your words and body never failed you to begin with. They saved you, and they certainly won't fail you now. Your reclamation carries with it endless possibilities for change, not just in thriving but also in prevention. Your heroism exists in the domain of individuality and mutuality; this is where you leave your legacy of pleasure, passion, and hope. I wish you well on the rest of your journey.

Your Allies and Resources Guide

Being an ally is more than just a label, it's a commitment to learn, to unlearn, to challenge, to change, and to sit in your discomfort. It's through that discomfort that change will happen.

—Tanya Compas

At its core, this book is for you and all survivors. Yet it also felt important for me to offer something to the people who love and care about you, those who often feel lost in knowing how to help. The following list is a collection of trusted references—some old, some new—for healing your mind, body, sexuality, and relationships. Many are specifically related to sexual trauma, while others offer solid advice on living happier, healthier, and sexier lives in the broader essence of sexual healing. Each of these resources will offer you and your partners, family, and friends a nonintrusive, sympathetic perspective for better understanding your process of recovery. They offer additional viewpoints and insights on key trauma, mental health, and sexual wellness principles, as well as self-care techniques and guidance for further validation rather than pathologization. Ideally, these resources will encourage your allies and supporters to tap into your resilience and mirror it, creating a bond where acceptance, authenticity, and honesty prospers.

MIND

Books

Brach, T. (2019). *Radical Compassion: Learning to Love Yourself and Your World with the Practice of RAIN*. New York, NY: Viking.

Brackett, M. (2020). *Permission to Feel: Unlocking the Power of Emotions to Help Our Kids, Ourselves, and Our Society Thrive*. New York, NY: Celadon Books.

Brown, B. (2012). *Daring Greatly: How the Courage to Be Vulnerable Transforms the Way We Live, Love, Parent, and Lead*. New York, NY: Avery.

Hicks-Wilson, D. (2020). *Small Cures*. Middletown, DE: Debra Hicks-Wilson.

Katie, B. (2008). *A Thousand Names for Joy: Living in Harmony with the Way Things Are*. New York, NY: Harmony.

Murthy, V. (2020). *Together: The Healing Power of Human Connection in a Sometimes Lonely World*. New York, NY: Harper Wave.

Wade, C. (2018). *Heart Talk: Poetic Wisdom for a Better Life*. New York, NY: Atria.

BODY

Books

Babbel, S. (2018). *Heal the Body, Heal the Mind: A Somatic Approach to Moving Beyond Trauma*. Oakland, CA: New Harbinger.

Braddock, C. (1997). *Body Voices: Using the Power of Breath, Sound, and Movement to Heal and Create New Boundaries*. Berkeley, CA: PageMill Press.

Dana, D. (2018). *The Polyvagal Theory in Therapy: Engaging the Rhythm of Regulation*. New York, NY: W. W. Norton & Company.

Porges, S. (2017). *The Pocket Guide to the Polyvagal Theory: The Transformative Power of Feeling Safe*. New York, NY: W. W. Norton & Company.

Rothschild, B. (2000). *The Body Remembers: The Psychophysiology of Trauma and Trauma Treatment*. New York, NY: W. W. Norton & Company, Inc.

Taylor, S. R. (2018). *The Body Is Not an Apology: The Power of Radical Self-Love*. Oakland, CA: Berrett-Koehler Publishers, Inc.

Van der Kolk, B. (2014). *The Body Keeps the Score: Brain, Mind, and Body in the Healing of Trauma*. New York, NY: Penguin Books.

Walker, P. (2013). *Complex PTSD: From Surviving to Thriving*. Lafayette, CA: Azure Coyote Publishing.

DISORDERED EATING

Books

Gay, R. (2018). *Hunger: A Memoir of (My) Body*. New York, NY: Harper Perennial.

Harrison, C. (2019). *Anti-Diet: Reclaim Your Time, Money, Well-Being, and Happiness Through Intuitive Eating*. New York, NY: Little, Brown Spark.

Knapp, C. (2003). *Appetites: Why Women Want*. New York, NY: Counterpoint.

Roth, G. (1992). *When Food Is Love: Exploring the Relationship Between Eating and Intimacy*. New York, NY: Penguin Books.

Schaefer, J. (2003). *Life Without Ed: How One Woman Declared Independence from Her Eating Disorder and How You Can Too.* New York, NY: McGraw-Hill Education.

Tribole, E., & Resch, E. (2020). *Intuitive Eating: A Revolutionary Anti-Diet Approach.* New York, NY: St. Martin's Press.

SEXUALITY

Sexual Trauma Prevention

End Rape On Campus (EROC)

Joyful Heart Foundation

National Alliance to End Sexual Violence

National Sexual Violence Resource Center

No More

Rape, Abuse & Incest National Network (RAINN)

SAFE

SafeBae

Trans Lifeline Peer Support

Transgender Law Center

Vday

Sex Education

Afrosexology

American Sexual Health Association

Dame Products (Swell blog)

Get Coral

Harvey Institute (The Six Principles of Sexual Health)

JuiceBox

Maven

MySexBio

OMGYes

Planned Parenthood (see chat feature, Roo, for answers to sexual heath questions)

Play Safe (STI testing and resources)

Scarleteen

Talk Tabu

Tantra4GayMen

Erotic Fiction

Bright Desire

Dipsea

Feminist Porn Awards

Himeros (for queer men)

Literotica

O'actually

Sssh

XConfessions (Erika Lust)

Books

Angel, K. (2021). *Tomorrow Sex Will Be Good Again: Women and Desire in the Age of Consent.* London, UK: Verso.

Bader, M. (2002). *Arousal: The Secret Logic of Sexual Fantasies.* New York, NY: Thomas Dunne Books.

Barker, M. J. (2016). *Queer: A Graphic History.* London, UK: Icon Books.

Bean, L., & Spade, D. (2018). *Written on the Body: Letters from Trans and Non-Binary Survivors of Sexual Assault & Domestic Violence.* London, UK: Jessica Kingsley Publishers.

Brotto, L. (2018). *Better Sex Through Mindfulness: How Women Can Cultivate Desire.* Vancouver, BC: Greystone Books.

Carrellas, B. (2007). *Urban Tantra: Sacred Sex for the Twenty-First Century.* Berkeley, CA: Celestial Arts.

Engle, G. (2019). *All the F*cking Mistakes: A Guide to Sex, Love, and Life.* New York, NY: St. Martin's Publishing Group.

Ensler, E. (2019). *The Apology.* New York, NY: Bloomsbury Publishing.

Goddard, A. J. (2015). *Woman on Fire: Nine Elements to Wake Up Your Erotic Energy, Personal Power, and Sexual Intelligence.* New York, NY: Avery.

Gunter, J. (2019). *The Vagina Bible: The Vulva and the Vagina—Separating Myth from Medicine.* New York, NY: Citadel Press.

Kay Klein, L. (2018). *Pure: Inside the Evangelical Movement That Shamed a Generation of Young Women and How I Broke Free.* New York, NY: Touchstone.

Kerner, I. (2004). *She Comes First: The Thinking Man's Guide to Pleasuring a Woman.* New York, NY: William Morrow Paperbacks.

Lehmiller, J. (2018). *Tell Me What You Want: The Science of Sexual Desire and How It Can Help You Improve Your Sex Life*. New York, NY: Da Capo Press.

Martin, W. (2018). *Untrue: Why Nearly Everything We Believe About Women, Lust, and Infidelity Is Wrong and How the New Science Can Set Us Free*. New York, NY: Little, Brown Spark.

Miller, C. (2019). *Know My Name*. New York, NY: Viking.

Mintz, L. (2018). *Becoming Cliterate: Why Orgasm Equality Matters—and How to Get It*. New York, NY: Harper One.

Morin, J. (1995). *The Erotic Mind: Unlocking the Inner Sources of Sexual Passion and Fulfillment*. New York, NY: Harper.

Nagoski, E. (2015). *Come as You Are: The Surprising New Science That Will Transform Your Sex Life*. New York, NY: Simon & Schuster.

Solomon, A. (2020). *Taking Sexy Back: How to Own Your Sexuality & Create the Relationships You Want*. Oakland, CA: New Harbinger.

Thomashauer, R. (2016). *Pussy: A Reclamation*. Carlsbad, CA: Hay House, Inc.

Viloria, H. (2017). *Born Both: An Intersex Life*. New York, NY: Hachette Books.

Walker, M. (2021). *Whole-Body Sex: Somatic Sex Therapy and the Lost Language of the Erotic Body*. New York, NY: Routledge.

Wichman, D. (2020). *Every Grain of Sand*. Nashville, TN: W. Brand Publishing.

Winston, S. (2010). *Women's Anatomy of Arousal: Secret Maps to Buried Treasure*. Kingston, NY: Mango Garden Press.

Zam, L. (2020). *The Pleasure Plan: One Women's Search for Sexual Healing*. Boca Raton, FL: Health Communications, Inc.

RELATIONSHIPS

Books

Finkle, E. (2017). *The All-or-Nothing Marriage: How the Best Marriages Work*. Boston, MA: Dutton.

Iasenza, S. (2020). *Transforming Sexual Narratives: A Relational Approach to Sex Therapy*. New York, NY: Routledge.

Johnson, S. (2013). *Love Sense: The Revolutionary New Science of Romantic Relationships*. New York, NY: Little, Brown, and Company.

Levine, A., & Heller, R. (2012). *Attached: The New Science of Adult Attachment and How It Can Help You Find—and Keep—Love*. New York, NY: TarcherPerigee.

Nelson, T. (2008). *Getting the Sex You Want: Shed Your Inhibitions and Reach New Heights of Passion Together*. Beverly, MA: Quiver Books.

Perel, E. (2007). *Mating in Captivity: Unlocking Erotic Intelligence*. New York, NY: Harper.

Roche, J. (2018). *Queer Sex: A Trans and Non-Binary Guide to Intimacy, Pleasure, and Relationships*. London, UK; Jessica Kingsley Publishers.

Snyder, S. (2018). *Love Worth Making: How to Have Ridiculously Great Sex in a Long-Lasting Relationship*. New York, NY: St. Martin's Press.

Solomon, A. (2017). *Loving Bravely: Twenty Lessons of Self-Discovery to Help You Get the Love You Want*. Oakland, CA: New Harbinger.

Tatkin, S. (2012). *Wired for Love: How Understanding Your Partner's Brain and Attachment Style Can Help You Defuse Conflict and Build a Secure Relationship*. Oakland, CA: New Harbinger.

The School of Life. (2020). *The Couple's Workbook*. London, UK: The School of Life.

FIND A THERAPIST

American Association of Sexuality Educators, Counselors and Therapists (AASECT)

Psychology Today

Rape, Abuse & Incest National Network (RAINN, locates local rape crisis centers and support groups)

Society for Sex Therapy and Research (SSTAR)

SUICIDE PREVENTION

American Foundation for Suicide Prevention

International Association for Suicide Prevention

National Suicide Prevention Line: (800) 273-8255

Trans Lifeline: US (877) 565-8860; Canada (877) 330-6366

The Trevor Project: (866) 488-7386

Acknowledgments

I started my career as a journalist almost three decades ago (in magazines, back when those were a thing), but always dreamed of writing a book. I've had nothing short of hundreds of ideas and almost as many starts and stops in origination. While this book has lived in me through my work as a psychologist for several years, the actual birth of it—words on pages—manifested quickly and with surprise, as the best births do, in my opinion. I never set out with the intention of working specifically with survivors of sexual trauma, though there is nothing unintentional or indeterminate about their place in my life now.

My earliest appreciation must go to another author whom I've never met, but whose book radically changed my life. Mark Salzman's *True Notebooks* taught me that words heal, and not just the people who read them. Cultures, societies, and systems can and will evolve when we let the most disenfranchised among us know we want to hear what they have to say. Thank you to Jill Gurr, founder of the nonprofit youth organization Create Now, for helping me find my first position teaching creative writing to incarcerated teens. The young women at California Youth Authority's Division for Juvenile Justice in Camarillo tearfully, candidly, and sometimes even hilariously inspired me to forge a path between writing and therapy. Your words were a catalyst for profound change in my life—I hope they served you well too.

It is not an overstatement to say this book would not have been possible without my teachers and clients, who were one and the same, at the Santa Barbara Rape Crisis Center. You laid the groundwork for reimagining what was possible in recovery from sexual trauma. Week after week you trusted me (an intern!) to walk with you on one of the most painful paths humans can endure. Your bravery lives in me and in this book. Thank you also to Marilyn Goldman, my clinical supervisor, who embodied equal parts wisdom and warmth.

Studying somatic psychology under the poetic tutelage of Edmond Knighton and Marti Glenn, among others, at the Santa Barbara Graduate Institute and The Chicago School of Professional Psychology, Los Angeles, cemented the body's centrality in the hurt and healing of sexual trauma. My mentor and fellow sex therapist, Suzanne Rapley, helped me connect pleasure to the entirety of emotional, relational, and sexual well-being.

More recently, a huge thank you to Esther Perel for your genuine interest in my work with survivors, and for believing I had something different and valuable to say. Your definition of Eros offered a critical accompaniment to the concept of thriving, which gave this book legs to stand on and a life force to breathe into. Alexandra Solomon, your warmth, support, generosity, and willingness to connect me with New Harbinger will forever be appreciated and repaid in kind to the next aspiring author.

To my talented editors, Jennye Garibaldi and Jennifer Holder, who have been fierce cheerleaders for this book since the opportunity was drafted. The entire team at New Harbinger, including Analis Souza and Mya Adriene Byrne, made a daunting process feel entirely doable. Your encouragement, insights, and, well, book smarts have been invaluable gifts. The early editing of this book was also made seamless through the critical eye of my research assistant, Willow Frederick. I have such appreciation for your willingness to take on everything I offered both cognitively and emotionally. I feel your heart in this book too.

To my friends who asked persistently about my progress with writing: Your patience with my process and deep belief in the possibilities for this book are irreplaceable. Only because you were sure I could do it, was I sure I could do it. Many of my clients offered encouragement and excitement about the evolution of this book too. Those of you from Santa Barbara to San Francisco, Long Beach, Los Angeles, New York City,

Portland, and New Jersey, you are in these pages. There would be no book without you.

With two small boys, Archer and Finn, a half-wild cat, Ninja, and my ever-amusing partner, Danny, home is always full of life (and noise). Add in a pandemic when no one can go anywhere, and the fun really began. I'm a person who needs quiet, and honestly a little space, to write. That would not have been possible without a team of supporters, coordinators, and wranglers, including my parents, Margie and Jerry Richmond, who colored, crafted, swam, canoed, and endured beestings and allergies over long summer weekends, as well as Brittany Marolakos and Bella Pagnotta, who said "yes" to every ask, and are more family than friends at this point. Danny, my heart and soul, you did not get many breaks. Please know I recognize that and appreciate you for thoughtfully picking up everything I couldn't. You have always been able to see the bigger, long-range picture so clearly. Thank you for supporting us to move toward a shared vision of a future that is full of grace, generosity, and love, not just for us and the people we love, but for all survivors too.

Endnotes

Introduction

1   Esther Perel, "Sessions Live 2019: In Search of Eros," November 9, 2019, livestream, https://sessions.estherperel.com.

2   Glennon Doyle, *Untamed* (New York, NY: The Dial Press, 2020), 141–142.

3   Hugh B. Urban, *Tantra: Sex, Secrecy, Politics, and Power in the Study of Religion* (Berkeley, CA: University of California Press, 2003), 25.

4   Rachel E. Morgan and Barbara A. Oudekerk, "Criminal Victimization, 2019," Homeland Security Digital Library, United States Bureau of Justice Statistics, published September 1, 2020, https://www.hsdl.org/?abstract&did=844138.

Chapter One

5   Esther Perel, *Mating in Captivity: Unlocking Erotic Intelligence* (New York, NY: Harper, 2007).

6   Thema Bryant-Davis, *Surviving Sexual Violence: A Guide to Recovery and Empowerment* (Lanham, MD: Rowman & Littlefield Publishers, Inc., 2011), 38.

7   "Crime in the United States 2016," Federal Bureau of Investigation, 2017, https://ucr.fbi.gov/crime-in-the-u.s/2016/crime-in-the-u.s.-2016/topic-pages/rape.

8   "Sexual Assault," RAINN (Rape, Abuse & Incest National Network), accessed March 13, 2021, https://www.rainn.org/articles/sexual-assault.

9   "Victims of Sexual Violence: Statistics," RAINN (Rape, Abuse & Incest National Network), accessed March 13, 2021, https://www.rainn.org/statistics/victims-sexual-violence.

10 Joanna Williams, *Women Vs Feminism: Why We All Need Liberating from the Gender Wars* (Bingley, UK: Emerald Publishing Limited, 2017).

11 "Sexual Abuse," American Psychological Association, accessed March 13, 2021, https://www.apa.org/topics/sexual-abuse.

12 Marije Stoltenborgh et al., "The Prevalence of Child Maltreatment Across the Globe: Review of a Series of Meta-Analyses," *Child Abuse Review* 24, no. 1 (2014): 37–50, https://doi.org/10.1002/car.2353.

13 "Perpetrators of Sexual Violence: Statistics," RAINN (Rape, Abuse & Incest National Network), accessed March 13, 2021, https://www.rainn.org/statistics/perpetrators-sexual-violence.

14 Bryant-Davis, *Surviving Sexual Violence* 38.

15 Jennifer L. Truman and Lynn Langton, "Criminal Victimization, 2013," U.S. Department of Justice, Bureau of Justice Statistics, 2013.

16 "Statistics," RAINN (Rape, Abuse and Incest National Network), accessed March 13, 2021, https://www.rainn.org/statistics.

17 "Violence Against Women," WHO (World Health Organization), revised March 9, 2021, https://www.who.int/news-room/fact-sheets/detail/violence-against-women.

18 "Perpetrators of Sexual Violence: Statistics," RAINN (Rape, Abuse & Incest National Network), accessed March 13, 2021, https://www.rainn.org/statistics/perpetrators-sexual-violence.

19 Holly Kearl, "The Facts Behind the #MeToo Movement: A National Study on Sexual Harassment and Assault," Stop Street Harassment, February 2018, 14–15, https://stopstreetharassment. org/our-work/nationalstudy/2018-national-sexual-abuse-report.

20 #MeToo was originally created by activist Tarana Burke in 2007 to reach survivors of sexual violence in marginalized communities. In the fall of 2017, actor Alyssa Milano reignited the hashtag on Twitter, and within forty-eight hours, there were nearly 1 million tweets. On Facebook, there were more than 12 million posts, comments, and reactions in less than twenty-four hours by 4.7 million users around the world who were sharing—many for the first time—that they too were survivors of unwanted sexual harassment, sexual abuse, and/or sexual assault.

21 "Working Definition of Sexual Pleasure," Global Advisory Board for Sexual Health and Wellbeing, 2016, https://www.gab-shw.org /our-work/working-definition-of-sexual-pleasure.

22 "World Report on Violence & Health," WHO (World Health Organization), October 3, 2002, https://www.who.int/violence _injury_prevention/violence/global_campaign/en/chap6.pdf.

23 "Key Terms and Phrases," RAINN (Rape, Abuse & Incest National Network), accessed March 13, 2021, https://www .rainn.org/articles/key-terms-and-phrases.

24 "Key Terms and Phrases," RAINN (Rape, Abuse & Incest National Network), accessed March 13, 2021, https://www .rainn.org/articles/key-terms-and-phrases.

Chapter Two

25 Emily Nagoski, *Come as You Are: The Surprising New Science That Will Transform Your Sex Life* (New York, NY: Simon & Schuster, 2015), 316.

26 Maurice Merleau-Ponty, *Phenomenology of Perception* (Paris, France: Editions Gallimard, 1945).

27 "Sexual Health," WHO (World Health Organization), 1975.

28 WHO (World Health Organization), "Defining Sexual Health: Report of a Technical Consultation on Sexual Health, 28–31 Janurary 2002, Geneva," 2006, https://www.who.int/repro ductivehealth/publications/sexual_health/defining_sexual _health.pdf.

29 Douglas Braun-Harvey and Michael Vigorito, *Treating Out of Control Sexual Behavior: Rethinking Sex Addiction* (New York, NY: Springer Publishing Company, 2015).

Chapter Three

30 Bessel van der Kolk, *The Body Keeps the Score: Brain, Mind, and Body in the Healing of Trauma* (New York, NY: Penguin Books, 2014), 27.

31 Susanne Babbel, *Heal the Body, Heal the Mind* (Oakland, CA: New Harbinger Publications, 2018), 33.

32 Babbel, *Heal the Body, Heal the Mind*, 34.

33 Maya Angelou, *I Know Why the Caged Bird Sings* (New York, NY: Random House, 1969), 1.

34 Stephen W. Porges, "Orienting in a Defensive World: Mammalian Modifications of Our Evolutionary Heritage: A Polyvagal Theory," *Psychophysiology* 32, no. 4 (1995): 301–318, http://doi.org/10.1111 /j.1469-8986.1995.tb01213.x.

35 Deb A. Dana, *The Polyvagal Theory in Therapy: Engaging the Rhythm of Regulation* (New York, NY: W. W. Norton & Company, 2018), 36.

36 Dana, *The Polyvagal Theory in Therapy*, 36.

37 Van der Kolk, *The Body Keeps the Score,* 67.

38 Van der Kolk, *The Body Keeps the Score,* 67.

39 Babette Rothschild, *The Body Remembers: The Psychophysiology of Trauma and Trauma Treatment* (New York, NY: W. W. Norton & Company, 2000), 155.

40 Perel, *Mating in Captivity.*

41 Marti Glenn, class lecture, Santa Barbara Graduate Institute, Santa Barbara, CA, October 2010.

42 Stella Resnick, *The Pleasure Zone: Why We Resist Good Feelings & How to Let Go and Be Happy* (Newburyport, MA: Conari Press, 1997), 23.

Chapter Four

43 Corinne Edwards, *Love Waits on Welcome: ...And Other Miracles* (Kalamazoo, MI: Steven J. Nash Publications, 1995), adapted from Gerald G. Jampolsky, *Love Is Letting Go of Fear* (New York, NY: Celestial Arts, 1979). This quote was later made famous by Lily Tomlin and other on-screen figures.

44 "Perpetrators of Sexual Violence: Statistics," RAINN (Rape, Abuse & Incest National Network), accessed March 13, 2021, https://www.rainn.org/statistics/perpetrators-sexual-violence.

45 Somatic psychology concept: source unknown.

46 Tara Brach, *Radical Compassion: Learning to Love Yourself and Your World with the Practice of RAIN* (New York, NY: Viking, 2019), 61.

47 Dana, *The Polyvagal Theory in Therapy,* 5.

48 Robert H. Howland, "Vagus Nerve Stimulation," *Current Behavioral Neuroscience Reports* 1, no. 2 (July 2014): 64–73, https://doi.org/10.1007/s40473-014-0010-5.

49 Van der Kolk, *The Body Keeps the Score,* 146.

50 Devon MacDermott, "Why Women Freeze During Sexual Assault," *Psychology Today,* May 3, 2018, https://www.psychologytoday.com/us/blog/modern-trauma/201805/why-women-freeze-during-sexual-assault.

51 MacDermott, "Why Women Freeze During Sexual Assault."

52 Walker, *Complex PTSD: From Surviving to Thriving* (Lafayette, CA: Azure Coyote Publishing, 2013).

Chapter Five

53 Hara Estroff Marano, "At a Loss," *Psychology Today,* June 19, 2020, https://www.psychologytoday.com/us/articles/202006/loss.

54 Byron Katie with Stephen Mitchell, *A Thousand Names for Joy: Living in Harmony with the Way Things Are* (New York, NY: Three Rivers Press, 2007), xiv.

55 Byron Katie with Stephen Mitchell, *Loving What Is: Four Questions That Can Change Your Life* (New York, NY: Harmony Books, 2002), 87.

56 Brené Brown, "Listening to Shame," filmed March 2, 2012, in Long Beach, CA, TED video, 20:22, https://www.ted.com/talks/brene_brown_listening_to_shame?language=en.

57 Brené Brown, *Daring Greatly: How the Courage to Be Vulnerable Transforms the Way We Live, Love, Parent, and Lead* (New York, NY: Avery, 2015), 69.

58 Brach, *Radical Compassion,* 73.

59 Michael Sieck, class lecture, Santa Barbara Graduate Institute, Santa Barbara, CA, 2010.

60 Brené Brown, *I Thought It Was Just Me (But It Isn't): Telling the Truth about Perfectionism, Inadequacy, and Power* (New York, NY: Gotham Books, 2008), 33.

61 Brené Brown, "Brené on Shame and Accountability," *Unlocking Us with Brené Brown,* podcast audio, July 1, 2020, https://brenebrown .com/podcast/brene-on-shame-and-accountability.

62 Brown, *I Thought It Was Just Me (But It Isn't),* 197.

63 Perel, *Mating in Captivity.*

Chapter Six

64 Peter A. Levine and Ann Frederick, *Waking the Tiger: Healing Trauma* (Berkeley, CA: North Atlantic Books, 1997), 32.

65 Virginia Woolf, *On Being Ill* (Ashfield, MA: Paris Press, 2002), 33.

66 Jonathan Bisson and Martin Andrew, "Psychological Treatment of Post-Traumatic Stress Disorder (PTSD)," *Cochrane Database System Reviews,* July 18, 2007, https://doi.org/10.1002/14651858.cd003388 .pub3.

67 Bryant-Davis, *Surviving Sexual Violence,* 71.

68 Levine and Frederick, *Waking the Tiger,* 32.

69 Mark G. Haviland, W. Louise Warren, and Matt L. Riggs, "An Observer Scale to Measure Alexithymia," *Psychosomatics* 41, no. 5 (2000): 385–392, https://doi.org/10.1176/appi.psy.41.5.385.

70 Mark Brackett, *Permission to Feel: Unlocking the Power of Emotions to Help Our Kids, Ourselves, and Our Society Thrive* (New York, NY: Celadon Books, 2019).

71 Ellen Bass and Laura Davis, *The Courage to Heal: A Guide for Women Survivors of Child Sexual Abuse* (New York, NY: Collins Living, 1988), 6–7.

72　Alice Miller, *The Body Never Lies: The Lingering Effects of Hurtful Parenting* (New York, NY: W. W. Norton & Company, 2005), 36.

73　Levine and Frederick, *Waking the Tiger,* 129.

74　Van der Kolk, *The Body Keeps the Score,* 67.

75　Gabor Maté, workshop presented at the Psychotherapy Networker Conference, Washington, DC, March 2019.

76　Jennifer Madowitz, Brittany Matheson, and June Liang, "The Relationship Between Eating Disorders and Sexual Trauma," *Eating and Weight Disorders* 20, no. 3 (2015): 281–293, https://doi.org/10.1007/s40519-015-0195-y.

77　Cynthia Price and Carole Hooven, "Interoceptive Awareness Skills for Emotion Regulation: Theory and Approach of Mindful Awareness in Body-Oriented Therapy (MABT)," *Frontiers in Psychology* 9 (2018): 798, https://doi.org/10.3389/fpsyg.2018.00798.

78　Joseph Critelli and Jenny Bivona, "Women's Erotic Rape Fantasies: An Evaluation of Theory and Research," *Journal of Sex Research* 45, no. 1 (2008): 57–70, https://doi.org/10.1080/00224490701808191.

79　Justin J. Lehmiller, *Tell Me What You Want: The Science of Sexual Desire and How It Can Help You Improve Your Sex Life* (New York, NY: Da Capo Press, 2018), 27.

80　Julia Camuso and Alessandra Rellini, "Sexual Fantasies and Sexual Arousal in Women with a History of Childhood Sexual Abuse," *Sexual and Relationship Therapy* 25, no. 3 (2010): 275–288, https://doi.org/10.1080/14681994.2010.494659.

81　Holly Richmond, "The Recovery of Sexual Health After Sexual Assault," ProQuest-CSA, LLC (2014): 35.

82　Mary Whitehouse, "The Tao of the Body," in *Bone, Breath and Gesture: Practices of Embodiment,* ed. Don Hanlon Johnson (Berkeley, CA: North Atlantic Books, 1995), 240–242.

83 Esther Perel, "About Me: My Story, Background, and Inspirations," EstherPerel.com, accessed March 13, 2021, https://www.esther perel.com/my-story.

84 Bass and Davis, *The Courage to Heal*, 388.

85 Amir Levine and Rachel Heller, *Attached: The New Science of Adult Attachment and How It Can Help You Find—and Keep—Love* (New York, NY: TarcherPerigee, 2010), 20.

86 Dan Siegel, *Mindsight: The New Science of Personal Transformation* (New York, NY: Bantam Books, 2011), xii.

87 Franklin D. Lewis, *Rumi—Past and Present, East and West: The Life, Teachings, and Poetry of Jalal al-Din Rumi* (London, UK: Oneworld Publications, 2000), 335.

Chapter Seven

88 Richmond, "The Recovery of Sexual Health After Sexual Assault."

89 Kaitlin A. Chivers-Wilson, "Sexual Assault and Posttraumatic Stress Disorder: A Review of the Biological, Psychological, and Sociological Factors and Treatments," *McGill Journal of Medicine* 9 (July 2006): 111–118.

90 Quoted in E. Alex Jung, "Michaela the Destroyer," *Vulture Magazine*, July 6, 2020, https://www.vulture.com/article/michaela -coel-i-may-destroy-you.html.

91 Christopher Rim, "Brené Brown and Marc Brackett on Emotional Intelligence During a Pandemic," *Forbes*, April 24, 2020, https:// www.forbes.com/sites/christopherrim/2020/04/24/bren-brown -and-marc-brackett-on-emotional-intelligence-during-a-pandemic /#42f37c69c0ae.

92 Gabor Maté, Psychotherapy Networker Conference, March 2019, Washington, DC.

93 Quoted in Mara B. Vernon, "We Must Talk About Hard Things," *Ripp Leadership Blog*, August 17, 2017, https://rippleadership.com/blog/we-must-talk-about-hard-things.

94 Quote by Maggie Kuhn, also attributed to Ruth Bader Ginsburg, date unknown, https://www.womenofthehall.org/inductee/maggie-kuhn.

95 Lisa Fritscher, "Coping with Anticipatory Anxiety," Verywell Mind, March 9, 2020, https://www.verywellmind.com/anticipatory-anxiety-2671554.

96 "Catastrophizing," *Psychology Today*, https://www.psychologytoday.com/us/basics/catastrophizing.

97 Suzanne Rapley, Santa Barbara, CA, 2009. Personal conversation.

98 Robin Sharma, "The 4 Fs of Change Resistance," RobinSharma.com, accessed September 25, 2020, https://www.robinsharma.com/article/the-4-fs-of-change-resistance.

99 Raymond Lloyd Richmond, *Boundaries: Protecting Yourself from Emotional Harm* (San Francisco, CA, 2018).

Chapter Eight

100 Alexandra Solomon, *Taking Sexy Back: How to Own Your Sexuality and Create the Relationships You Want* (Oakland, CA: New Harbinger Publications, 2020), 4.

101 Nagoski, *Come as You Are*, 185.

102 Wendy Maltz, *The Sexual Healing Journey: A Guide for Survivors of Sexual Abuse* (New York, NY: HarperCollins Publishers, 2001), 104.

103 Sonya Renee Taylor, *The Body Is Not an Apology* (Oakland, CA: Berrett-Koehler Publishers, Inc., 2018), 3.

104 Laura Zam, *The Pleasure Plan: One Woman's Search for Sexual Healing* (Boca Raton, FL: Health Communications Inc., 2020), 240.

105 Katherine Rowland, *The Pleasure Gap* (New York, NY: Seal Press, 2020), 123.

106 Nagoski, *Come as You Are*, 193.

107 Sheri Winston, *Women's Anatomy of Arousal: Secret Map to Buried Treasure* (Kingston, NY: Mango Garden Press, 2010), 13.

108 @cyndi_darnell, Instagram, October 2, 2020.

109 Staci Haines, *Healing Sex: A Mind-Body Approach to Healing Sexual Trauma* (San Francisco, CA: Cleis Press Inc., 2007), 89.

110 Gigi Engle, *All the F*cking Mistakes* (New York, NY: St. Martin's Griffin, 2019), 67.

Chapter Nine

111 Stephen Porges, *The Pocket Guide to the Polyvagal Theory: The Trans-formative Power of Feeling Safe* (New York, NY: W. W. Norton & Company, 2017).

112 Levine and Heller, *Attached*, 21.

113 Brené Brown, *The Gifts of Imperfection* (Center City, MN: Hazelden Publishing, 2010), 5.

114 Richmond, "The Recovery of Sexual Health After Sexual Assault"; Marci Littlefield and Tamara Leech, "Social Support and Resilience in the Aftermath of Sexual Assault: Suggestions across Life Course, Gender, and Racial Groups," in Bryant-Davis, *Surviving Sexual Violence*, 296–317; Richard Brown and Patricia Gerbarg, "Mind-Body Practices for Recovery from Sexual Trauma," in Bryant-Davis, *Surviving Sexual Violence*, 199–216.

115 Barbara Keesling, *Sexual Healing: The Complete Guide to Overcoming Common Sexual Problems* (Alameda, CA: Hunter House, 2006), 31.

116 John Gottman and Julie Gottman, *The Science of Couples and Family Therapy: Behind the Scenes at the Love Lab* (New York, NY: W. W. Norton & Company, 2018), 36.

117 Winston, *Women's Anatomy of Arousal*, 48.

118 Dawn Cartwright, "Sex Magic, Week 6: Magnetism & Receptivity," Chandra Bidu Tantra Institute, 2012, http://www .mynewsletterbuilder.com/email/newsletter/1411698311.

119 Barbara Carrellas, *Urban Tantra: Sacred Sex for the Twenty-First Century* (New York, NY: Celestial Arts, 2007), 124.

120 "Sensate Focus," Cornell Health, October 18, 2019, adapted from William H. Masters, Virginia E. Johnson, and Robert C. Kolodny, *Heterosexuality* (New York, NY: Harper Collins, 1994), https:// health.cornell.edu/sites/health/files/pdf-library/sensate-focus.pdf.

121 "Sensate Focus," Cornell Health.

122 Della Hicks-Wilson, *Small Cures* (London, UK: Della Hicks-Wilson, 2020), 144.

Chapter Ten

123 Finn Deerhart, "Porn and Racism: Uncovering Our Broken Relationships to Power," FinnDeerhart.com, June 27, 2020, https://mailchi.mp/453adfcdbe0c/porn-racism-uncovering-our -broken-relationships-to-power.

124 Wednesday Martin, *Untrue: Why Nearly Everything We Believe About Women, Lust, and Infidelity Is Wrong and How the New Science Can Set Us Free* (New York, NY: Little, Brown Spark, 2018), 12.

125 Nazanin Moali, "Understanding—and Not Fearing—Your Sexual Fantasies," Oasis2Care.com, November 18, 2020, https://oasis2care .com/sexuality/understanding-and-not-fearing-your-sexual-fantasies.

126 Ian Kerner, *She Comes First: The Thinking Man's Guide to Pleasuring a Woman* (New York, NY: Collins, 2004), 89.

127 Lehmiller, *Tell Me What You Want.*

128 Tammy Nelson, *Getting the Sex You Want: Shed Your Inhibitions and Reach New Heights of Passion Together* (Beverly, MA: Quiver, 2008), 115.

129 Perel, *Mating in Captivity,* 167.

130 Esther Perel and Mary Alice Miller, "Why Do Sexual Taboos Make Up Our Sexual Fantasies?" EstherPerel.com, July 2020, https://estherperel.com/blog/sexual-taboos-sexual-fantasy.

131 Sigal Samuel, "How to Make This Winter Not Totally Suck, According to Psychologists," *Vox,* February 22, 2020, https://www .vox.com/future-perfect/2020/10/14/21508422/winter-dread-covid -19-pandemic-happiness-psychology.

Conclusion

132 "False Reporting Overview," National Sexual Violence Resource Center, 2012, https://www.nsvrc.org/sites/default/files/Publications _NSVRC_Overview_False-Reporting.pdf.

133 Gabor Maté, *In the Realm of Hungry Ghosts: Close Encounters with Addiction* (Berkeley, CA: North Atlantic Books, 2008).

134 David P. Wichman and Heather Ebert, *Every Grain of Sand: A Memoir* (Nashville, TN: W. Brand Publishing, 2020), 11.

135 Quoted in E. Alex Jung, "Michaela the Destroyer," *Vulture Magazine,* July 6, 2020, https://www.vulture.com/article/michaela -coel-i-may-destroy-you.html.

136 #MeToo was originally created by activist Tarana Burke in 2007 to reach survivors of sexual violence in underprivileged communities. In the fall of 2017, actress Alyssa Milano reignited the hashtag on Twitter, and within forty-eight hours, there were nearly 1 million tweets. On Facebook, there were more than 12 million posts, comments, and reactions in less than twenty-four hours by 4.7 million users around the world who were sharing, many for the first time, that they too were survivors of unwanted sexual harassment, sexual abuse, and/or sexual assault.

137 The #TimesUp movement was founded in Hollywood in January 2018 by a group of more than 300 women, as an extension of the #MeToo movement. While #MeToo is focused on conversation and community healing in relation to all kinds of sexual assault, #TimesUp is an organization focused on creating workplaces for women free of sexual assault, harassment, and discrimination.

138 Chanel Miller, *Know My Name: A Memoir* (New York, NY: Viking, 2019), 328.

139 Neil McArthur, "Is Lying to Get Laid a Form of Sexual Assault?" *Vice*, September 4, 2016, https://www.vice.com/en/article/4w5w7g/is-lying-to-get-laid-a-form-of-sexual-assault.

140 Maté, *In the Realm of Hungry Ghosts*, xxix.

Holly Richmond, PhD, is a somatic psychotherapist, certified sex therapist, and licensed marriage and family therapist. She is a frequent contributor to publications and media outlets on the intersection of psychology and sexuality, specializing in the treatment of survivors and the recovery of sexual health after trauma.

Foreword writer **Alexandra H. Solomon, PhD,** is clinical assistant professor in the department of psychology at Northwestern University, a licensed clinical psychologist at The Family Institute at Northwestern University, and author of *Loving Bravely.*

MORE BOOKS from
NEW HARBINGER PUBLICATIONS

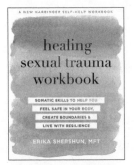
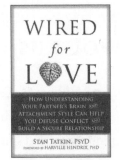
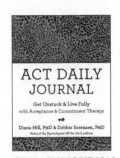
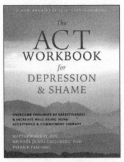
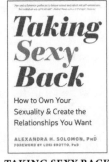
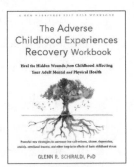